THE NHS:
A PICTURE OF HEALTH?

The NHS:
A Picture of Health?

Steve Iliffe

LAWRENCE AND WISHART
LONDON

Lawrence & Wishart Limited
39 Museum Street
London WC1A 1LQ

First published 1983

Photoset in North Wales by
Derek Doyle & Associates, Mold, Clwyd
Printed and bound in Great Britain by
The Camelot Press Ltd, Southampton

Contents

Figures

Preface

This is not a history book, but an attempt to understand the history of the National Health Service, and to predict its possible futures. The parts played by organised labour, by professionals and by political parties in the creation of the NHS are sometimes clear, sometimes obscure. I hope this account makes those parts easier to understand by describing their important relationships and alliances: between labour and professionalism; between professionals and capital; and between Fabian and Conservative ideas about the state and its powers.

It was written for everyone concerned with the politics of health, especially those who know that major changes are imminent and necessary, and who want to develop new relationships, new alliances and new working practices. This book cannot solve their problems, but perhaps it may help to clarify them.

It starts from the illnesses, disabilities, pain and fear that mark everyday life, and that are the proper objects of health care. I hope it is an antidote to the conventional radicalism that dismisses health care and medicine as commercial conspiracies or oppressive power relations, designed simply to keep people in their place. However much truth there is in these views (and there is enough), they do not start at or stay with the urgency of people's experiences. Sociology is indifferent to the lived reality of disease and disability, and imagines that illness has disappeared just because its graphs point downwards. The radicalism born of sociology shares that indifference and ultimately succumbs to professionalism, however patriarchal and controlling it may be. Perhaps the fundamental issue is: how can professionalism be changed?

Many people have have helped me with this book, through their written work or through hours of discussion over many years. I have learned a lot from Jane Bernal, Mick Carpenter,

Kate Gardner, Adrian Hastings, Keith Jerrome, Sue Lewis, Alison Macfarlane, the Radical Nurses Group, John Robson, Gerry Shulman, Cyril Taylor, Julian Tudor Hart and the late Alistair Wilson. Pat Conroy reminded me about doubt and ambiguity, throughout the writing. Michel Coleman helped me with references, more than he realises. Mrs Eugenia Robbin-Coker unscrambled tapes, and Eileen Ferrari deciphered my scrawl, to produce impressive manuscripts. A lot of people tolerated my variable temper during the writing of this book, but Uschi Haug weathered the worst of it.

Steve Iliffe
July 1983

CHAPTER 1

'The Jewel in Labour's Crown'

In 1917 it was safer to be a soldier on the Western Front than to be born in England. For every nine soldiers killed in France twelve babies died within their first year of life, in Britain. The infant casualty rate was 1,000 per week.

Our television documentaries present us with history as drama. Corpses hanging on barbed wire, wavering lines of grey figures advancing into the machine-guns, perhaps the red flags of the Bolshevik Revolution – these are the images of 1917. What happened to that other drama, the greater massacre of new born children, their mothers suffering from 'childbed fever', their fathers' health undermined in factory work or on the land? It has been relegated to history books, to statistical tables, and to the fading folk memory of those generations. Yet the experience of babies lost and families decimated powered the campaign for healthier working and living conditions, and for better medical services, throughout the first half of the twentieth century. The cause of Labour grew upon such experience, and a whole new society emerged from the struggle for change. Now we learn the history of our health services as a dry list of legislative reforms, or as a cascade of scientific advances. The living substance of that history, and its relationship to the rise of a labour movement, has been filleted, politely but firmly, from commonplace understanding.

Health politics begins with the Industrial Revolution. Rapid industrialisation at the beginning of the 19th century led to migration of huge numbers of people from the countryside into the new cities. In the ten years from 1821 the population of Manchester and Salford rose by 47%, whilst Bradford increased it civic population by 78% and West Bromwich by 60%. The housing hastily thrown up for the new working class was poor quality, cramped in huddles around the factories, deprived of adequate clean water supplies, and dependent on sanitation systems developed in medieval villages. The cities became reservoirs of disease and death. The nation's death rate began to rise after 1816, having fallen in the previous period. The death rate in country districts in the 1830s was about 18 per thousand compared with an average rate of 26 per thousand in the towns and cities. The average age of death in Manchester in the early part of the 19th century was 38 years for the upper middle class, but 17 years for the labouring class. In Liverpool the same figures were 35 years for the upper middle class and 15 years for the labouring class. Disease and death came from infections (like tuberculosis, typhus and diphtheria), from overwork in dangerous conditions, and from the consequences of alcoholism and syphilis. Tuberculosis was the main killer within the working population, causing between one third and one fifth of deaths during the Industrial Revolution. It was an infection that followed closely behind malnutrition, exhaustion and overcrowding. It concentrated in the new slums, and much less frequently selected more affluent victims.

Cholera, Syndicalism and Chartism

From the pain, misery and despair of the cities, three horrors emerge to fight the new breed of industrialists – cholera, syndicalism, and Chartism. All emerged from the slums and threatened to harm the established order. Four major cholera epidemics occurred in the 19th century, in 1831-32, 1848-49, 1853-54, and 1865-66. Cholera was not a major contributor to the high death rates in industrial Britain, in the long term. But it had a dramatic impact on the population, because it spread via water supplies and poor hygiene. Whilst the affluent did not suffer from overcrowding and malnutrition, they did share water supplies and similar standards of hygiene with the poor. Unlike tuberculosis, cholera did not respect wealth.

The second horror was syndicalism. Trade unions had grown as subversive organisations since the Jacobin agitation at the beginning of the century. They had been harrassed by police pressure and, at times, open military terror, and had developed their own counter-terror. Unrest in the labouring classes came to a head with the formation of the Grand National Consolidated Trades Union in 1834. This huge union recruited half a million members, a membership unimaginable before 1834, and soon became involved in a massive strike wave. The government counter-attacked, selecting for its attack trade union organisation in the Dorset village of Tolpuddle. The GNCTU launched their defence campaign for the Tolpuddle Martyrs and led a vast demonstration of trade unionists, between 100,000 and 200,000 in total, through London. This was the first great demonstration of working class power, and it had the same impact (on the affluent) as a cholera epidemic. The GNCTU did not survive its internal problems after the Tolpuddle case, but a new political movement called Chartism grew from the craft unions. Between 1837 and 1848 Chartism mobilised political feeling within the working population, and at one point (in 1839) came close to organizing an armed insurrection.

The responses to syndicalism and Chartism were political and repressive, but the government also realised that it needed to change social conditions to reduce the threat to established power. It began by dealing with the problem that had the highest priority for the new industrialist class, and for the affluent generally. Cholera. A central Board of Health was established in 1831, and a Cholera Prevention Act passed in 1832, in an attempt to control disease outbreaks. Local Boards of Health were formed in England and Scotland to implement the new policy. The Poor Law, which distributed meagre relief to the destitute, was reformed. Compulsory unification of parishes into Poor Law Unions with central asylums, work houses and orphanages, occurred. Specialised hospitals were proposed, but not built. A National Poor Law Commission to coordinate the operation of this streamlined Poor Law system was established. The architect of Poor Law Reform, Edwin Chadwick, investigated deaths from infectious diseases, and related death and disease incidence to overcrowding. He demonstrated that average age of death could be related to class: 43 years for the gentry; 30 years for tradesmen; 22 years for labourers. He found that in 1840, 100,000 children had been orphaned, and 27,000 women widowed through the death of the family bread-winner from infectious disease. He also pointed out the danger of short life expectancy in the labouring classes. Disease thinned the ranks of higher age groups, leaving a young, passionate and politically volatile population prone to 'extremist' solutions. His biographer said that Chadwick 'drew his respectable hearers to the edge of the pit and bade them observe the monsters they were breeding beneath their feet.'

What they saw was enough. The Public Health movement began, and ran on into the next century. Medical Offices of Health, Sanitary Acts, salaried doctors and local Boards of Health followed thick and fast. They made little impression on cholera, however, since they did not tackle the main cause – infected water supplies. That had to wait until after the third great Cholera epidemic, in 1853-54, and took shape in the Public Health Acts of 1858 and 1859. Water supplies were improved and regulated, though not without a battle with the private water companies. Sewage disposal methods that were largely unchanged from medieval times were abandoned in favour of closed drainage systems. More legislation was introduced in 1866 (Sanitary Act), 1867 (Factory and Workshop Acts), 1868 (the Torrens Act controlling the quality of housing) and 1871 (Vaccination Act).

Trade Unionism, TB and the Poor Law

This flurry of reforms occurred as British industry itself changed. By the end of the 1840s British capital had broken all the barriers to its growth, including the Chartist movement. Unprecedented industrial and commercial expansion returned profits at rates of thousands per cent. Falling raw material costs and cheap imports of food allowed profitability to increase at the same time as wages rose. Industrial production became more complex and technical. Unskilled labour, easily replaced by migration from the countryside in the earlier part of the century, gave way to skilled labour. A fitter, more knowledgeable and more reliable workforce was needed. Wages began to rise in the 1860s, and continued to do so (with one brief interlude) until the turn of the century. Food availability changed, with a higher meat and vegetable consumption within the working class. Death rates amongst adults began to fall from 1870 onwards. Trade unionism, from 1850, to 1880, concentrated on the 'pompous trades and proud mechanics', and their slogans were 'defence not defiance' and 'a fair day's pay for a fair day's work'. The ruthless exploitation of labour in the first phase of industrialisation seemed to be ending, and with it the wholesale squandering of people's health.

Sadly, the change was less than it appeared. The important

were preserved, but the expendable were expended as before. A survey of 'hurtful or hurtfully conducted occupations' in 1863 revealed how small cottage industries were as hazardous to their workers as were the great factories. Concurrent research showed that malnutrition was common-place, often because of the ignorance about food as much as through low purchasing power. Overcrowding was appalling, particularly in the mining areas of the North and the Midlands. One researcher had found 300 cases where families occupying one room took in lodgers to supplement their income. Starvation and drugging with opium were the two most commons causes of infant deaths in some rural areas. Malaria, once the cause of many childhood deaths, had been eradicated by the same land drainage that allowed women workers to be used in agriculture, at low wages, without access to child-care. Every year 'consumption' (tuberculosis of the lung) killed more people than small-pox, scarlet fever, measles, whooping-cough and typhus put together. Nearly four in every thousand died from tuberculosis in 1851. It took 50 years for the death rate from TB to fall to just under two per thousand.

The rate of change in provisions for health slowed down once the important sections of the population were protected, and political stability achieved. Emphasis changed from public health measures to medical intervention. For most of the people, most of the time, 19th century medicine had little to offer. It was an empirical art, aimed more at consoling the ill than at curing them. There were remedies for specific complaints, and both educated physicians and humble apothecaries could treat constipation, relieve pain and steady the pulse with digitalis, a herbal treatment prepared from foxgloves. Curing cholera, TB, diphtheria or any other serious infection (apart from small pox, against which some protection could be given) was beyond medical art. Surgery was nasty, bloody, brutal and short.

By 1900 medicine had gained a scientific basis, even though it retained a super-structure of priestcraft and superstition. Anaesthesia, of a crude kind, became available in mid-century, and gave surgeons precious time to work. Preventing wound infection after surgery became feasible by the 1870s, and death from complications of surgery became a less frequent event. Brain, chest and abdominal surgery became possible by the turn of the century.

The response from the working class was to organise pre-paid medical care for itself. Trade union funds in the quiet days of 1850-80 were used to finance a wide range of benefits, and the unions of 'pompous trades and proud mechanics' came to function as Trades Friendly Societies. The trade unions did not invent the idea of collecting for benefit. They borrowed it from the medical clubs, friendly societies and mutual benefit societies that had first developed at the end of the 18th century. These were usually local organisations, some of which went on to become major national institutions, collecting money from the 'provident' on a weekly basis and giving benefits in return. Death grants, unemployment, superannuation and ultimately sickness benefits were built up via the trade unions subscriptions. Some trade unions began to emulate the medical club, paying doctors to care for their members. The doctors often did little of medical value, but they could certify sickness, try to deal with the endless string of illnesses, and point the seriously ill towards treatment that was potentially effective. This system of pre-paid medical care was to shape the future of health services for over a century, generating the 'panel system' and later the general practioner's independent contract with the National Health Service.

The alternatives to these kinds of social provisions were grim. Doctors employed by the parish, under the provisions of the Poor Law, would attend only to the utterly destitute. For the poor serious illness meant a move into the hated Workhouse, where conditions were disgusting, or into a separate Poor Law Infirmary, where at least there may have been rudimentary nursing care. The trade unions' logic in organising some kind of access to marginally better quality care was unchallengeable.

All this was threatened by a down-turn in the economy. Britain's industrial and trading monopoly was challenged towards the end of the century, principally by Germany. Falling profits led to increased prices and slower wage rises. Relative industrial harmony gave way to renewed conflict, and a transformation of the trade union movement. 'New Unionism' emerged in the 1880s, militant and socialist in character, and challenged the employers and their political system. The 'New Unionism' was not interested in sickness benefits and medical clubs – it began to talk about state provision, and, worse still, about a new state. A new party of Labour was formed in 1900 to challenge the dominant Liberals. A trade union offensive began in 1910 and lasted till the beginning of the long-threatened war with Germany. It was at this point that a new round of social reforms was born, as all else appeared ready to collapse.

1911 – The Beginnings of the NHS?

In 1911 the Liberal Prime Minister, Lloyd George, introduced the National Health Insurance Act. This created the 'Panel System', under which employed working men and some of the middle classes with low incomes, could receive free medical care from general practitioners, and also free treatment for tuberculosis. The 'Panel' was simply an extension of the earlier club system, with a much wider commercial involvement. The old friendly societies were still empowered to collect National Health Insurance (NHI) contributions, but insurance companies and trade unions were also included in the system as collectors. Subscriptions raised under the NHI Act were used to fund the free medical care, and also to provide sickness benefit. This sickness benefit stopped when the working person retired, but the medical benefits continued. With modifications the Panel System continued until 1948, starting with an eligible population of 15 million in 1913 and rising to over 25 million in the mid 1940s, an increase from one third to one half of the population. The NHI Act excluded the dependents of insured workers, most of those who were unemployed, the majority of those in non-manual occupations, and all those needing treatment in hospitals.

The 1911 Reform is seen by some as the beginnings of the National Health Service in Britain, and by others as evidence that the state was only concerned with medical preparations for the coming war with Germany. Those views caricature a complex set of reasons for introducing reform within health care. The panel system was no great innovation. It was merely the nationalisation of an existing form of health care provision. It established the principles of government subsidy of medical services, but left the organisation of those services to a variety of professional and commercial interests. The job of implementing the 1911 Act could have been given to local government, but instead it was allocated to a cumbersome machinery of Insurance Committees which contained representatives from friendly societies, commercial insurance agencies and trade unions. Apart from sickness benefit, the main problems in the population's health were ignored by the Act: adequate maternity care; provision for child care; and expansion of the TB sanatoria. The chief beneficiaries of the Act must have the doctors already enrolled in the club system, for they achieved both an increase in income and freedom from club controls. The amount of money that the general practitioners received per patient almost doubled with NHI, and they were no longer required to supply drugs at their own expense for insured persons. Prescriptions were dealt with by chemists, who in turn were paid directly by the state. No longer were the doctors subject to appointment and dismissal by club committees. General practitioners could decide whether they wished to work for the NHI system or not. All they had to do was to register with the Insurance Committee and build up their lists of panel patients to any size that they thought fit. Private practice was not interferred with in any way, and the panel system became a way of developing a large private practice while still earning a reasonable income.

The political significance of the 1911 Act lay in the allies that it created for the Liberal government. The Liberals faced unprecedented labour agitation, watched the rise of the Labour Party that was later to replace it, and noted the growing demands for state-organised medical care. To retain control of the working class vote and undermine the influence of the new Labour Party, the Liberals had to give the organised working class its due. They also had to think of the impending war with Germany. The poor physical health of soldiers in the Boer War had certainly frightened the military and the politicians. However there was no reason to think that the reforms introduced in 1911 could resolve this problem in time, for the ill health of the working population stemmed from social problems, rather than lack of medical services. Had the Liberals paid attention to levels of nutrition, the quality of housing, work-safety, and possibly made provisions for better control of infectious diseases like tuberculosis, they could have argued that the 1911 reform was intended to produce a healthier population. The Liberal need was a different one, however. They had to make the working population believe that the coming war with Germany was worth fighting, because at the end of it there would be substantial social change that would benefit the whole population. Gaining acceptance of war ambitions was vital given the commitments of the Socialist and Labour Parties throughout Europe to a peace policy prior to 1914. With this longer term perspective, the Liberals found a second reason for initiating social reform. Finally, they had another enemy nearer home. The Conservatives were threatening to promote civil war in Ireland if the issue of Home Rule proceeded. Again the Liberals needed to buy allies, not against Germany this time, but against the Conservatives and Unionists, in case of major conflict over Irish Home Rule. Lloyd George hoped that, with the 1911 NHI Act, the Liberals could satisfy the demands of organised labour, rob the Labour Party of a contentious issue, and also meet the needs of the growing and increasingly vociferous medical profession. Improving the health of the industrial workforce, and of the potential conscript army, were not realisable goals, and did not become so until after the First World War.

War and a New Ministry

The war against Germany and its allies had a dramatic impact on the politics of health. The population in Britain did support the war effort, but as the casualty lists grew and the gains diminished, the demand for a better society after the war became stronger and more widespread. In the field of medicine the war fuelled the campaign for social change. Medical techniques were perfected or introduced, and further great advances seemed imminent. Surgery rapidly became a skilled art, with many surgeons gaining experience in chest, abdomen and skull surgery on a wide scale. Blood transfusion was introduced at the Battle of Cambrai in 1917. Army medical services showed that by careful planning it was possible to deal, after a fashion, with large numbers of injured soldiers, screening the injured for those who could best be helped, and passing the cases suitable for further treatment to specialist units. As the war ended the public debate about reforming medical services re-opened. The issue became one of providing centralised, efficient state-run services. The Liberals, re-elected in 1918 but faced with a signifcant Labour presence in the new Parliament, had to meet this demand for efficiency and effectiveness. Their problem was that of finding a solution that would satisfy the advocates of state control while preserving professional power and commercial interests within the medical services. A Ministry of Health was established in 1919, to initiate the process of centralisation and planning. The two driving forces behind the creation of the Ministry, and the general movement for state-run services, were the trade unions and the women's organisations. The trade unions particularly wanted national control of the hospitals run by charitable organisations. The women's organisations had tended to concentrate on the question of suffrage, but extended their interests to other fields, particularly after the vote had been achieved for women over 30 years, in 1918. The women's movement saw government co-ordination of medical care as a pre-condition for extension of services to women and their families.Challenged by a plan for a national health service, run by local government and staffed by salaried doctors (produced by the Socialist Medical Association's forerunner, the State Medical Services Association), the Liberals responded with the Dawson Report in 1920. Lord Dawson was the first Minister of Health in the Lloyd George Government, and his Report accepted some of the ideas and terminology of the SMSA plan but rejected the principles of state control, salaried doctors and integration of preventive and curative services. Instead 'co-ordination' of existing facilities was advocated, with ample provision for private practice as an antidote to the 'mediocrity' that allegedly followed salaries and excess control. Neither the Dawson Report nor the SMSA proposals survived the decline in labour militancy that occured in the late 1920s, although both were to re-appear in updated forms at the next crisis-point, over twenty years later.

From the formation of the Ministry of Health in 1919, to the creation of the NHS in 1948, women and labour formed a coalition of interests aiming to expand and organise a jumble of medical services run by central and local government, by charitable organisations, by insurance committees, and through the Poor Law. At the end of the First World War a working class family could receive medical care from as many as 9 different doctors working under 5 different organisations. The working man would see his panel doctor for all illnesses apart from tuberculosis. His wife, if she was insured, would see the same panel doctor for her illnesses, except for tuberculosis and problems in child-birth. If she was not insured then she could see a private doctor (if she could afford it) or, if she was too poor, a parish doctor (provided under Poor Law Regulations) or a doctor from a medical charity. During pregnancy she would use the municipal maternity service, and at her confinement would be attended by a midwife or a doctor from this service. Any member of the family who contracted tuberculosis would receive treatment from a local government tuberculosis doctor. Infants and children up to school age would be looked after by the maternity centre doctor. After they had gone to school they would be attended for 'school diseases' by the school medical officer, and by a private doctor (who was probably the family's panel doctor too) when they were too ill to go to school. After school age and up to 16 they would use the private doctor, but after 16 they would be able to see the same doctor under the panel system. Separate staffs were organised to administer each service, with little effort at co-ordination. The Poor Law medical services effectively overlapped with municipal care, but two systems of administration were used to run them, and entirely independent networks of medical officers were organised. During the 1920s this complexity was made worse by the appointment of specialist medical officers to deal with particular diseases – tuberculosis, measles, diseases associated with maternity, and venereal diseases.

The hospital system was equally chaotic. Some hospitals were voluntary hospitals, run by charities. Others were private nursing homes or private cottage hospitals, used by those who could afford to pay their fees. Municipalities ran their own hospitals, clinics and sanatoria, and there were also Poor Law hospitals still in existence. The quality and quantity of hospitals in any area, and the services that they provided, depended on the interests shown in them by local government, by charitable organisation and by enthusiastic reformers working within them. Whilst new services were introduced throughout the twenties and thirties, particularly in the fields of maternity care and child-care, the administrative chaos means that new developments in science could not be applied in any systematic and effective way. For example, immunisation against diphtheria became possible in 1913. The Ministry of Health recommended its general use in 1922, and this was reinforced by a report from the Medical Research Council in 1927. All local authorities were urged to start mass immunisation campaigns, but very little happened.

From 1922-1940 about 3,000 children a year continued to die from this wholly preventable disease. Most medical effort went into dealing with individually presented symptoms. The emphasis was on making early diagnosis of the disease using throat swabs, treating the affected person with an antidote, and admitting him or her to the diphtheria ward in a hospital. When the child became to ill to breathe because the upper part of the throat was blocked, an emergency tracheotomy – an artificial opening in the neck to allow breathing – was made. A national immunisation campaign began, after much delay, in 1940, and death rates from diphtheria dropped dramatically. Had the medical services been geared towards preventive care, rather than heroic cures, perhaps 30,000 lives could have been extended.

The same sad story aplies to other infectious diseases. Nearly 2,000 children died each year from whooping cough. Tuberculosis killed between 30,000 and 40,000 people a year, mostly young people between the ages of 15 and 25. Tuberculosis attacked the poorer sections of the population, just as it had done in the 19th century. During the worst years of the depression in the 1930s the death rates from tuberculosis in the worst hit areas of the country, the North East and South Wales, were twice the rate in England and Wales as a whole. Even where there had been substantial improvements since the turn of century, as in the infant death rate, there were wide disparities between different regions, reflecting poverty and high unemployment. Death rates were much higher for all conditions in Scotland, the North of England and in Wales than they were for most of the South of England. In 1935 the infant death rate was only 42 per thousand live births in the Home Counties, but it was 63 in Glamorgan, 76 in Durham, 77 in Scotland, 92 in Sunderland and 114 in Jarrow.

Wealth, or the lack of it, determined standards of health, paterns of illness, and the use of medical services. The use of dental services demonstrated the huge differences within the population. The more affluent would attend the dentist regularly, paying fees for each visit, but expecting to have their teeth kept in good order. For the majority of the working population, bad teeth were one of the normal misfortunes of life. A trip to the dentist was called for when the toothache became unbearable, and they would then expect to have the tooth pulled out. Almost inevitably, by the time they reached the dentist extraction was usually the only remedy. Even this cost money because the NHI benefit usually did not extend to dental care. The need for artificial dentures in a poor home was a major financial calamity.

Maternity care for working women was provided mainly by local midwives, and to a lesser extent by municipal doctors. The fee charged by midwives depended on the locality, or on the financial position of the pregnant woman and her family. Many midwives were as poor as the people they served, and did not receive appropriate training or technical support. Maternal mortality began to rise in the early 1930s. At least half of the deaths of mothers in childbirth were directly preventable; the four primary avoidable causes were: lack of ante-natal care; errors of judgement or treatment by doctors or midwives; lack of reasonable facilities for medical care; and negligence by the patients. Improvements in maternity services were important issues for women's organisations throughout the inter-war period, despite all the attempts to make piecemeal changes in medical services for women and their families.

Crisis, War and the Birth of the NHS

As the Second World War approached a combination of factors made another round of social reform inevitable. The first drugs effective against infections were introduced, starting with Salvarsan, which could be used to cure syphilis. 'Sulfa Drugs' were introduced in the late 1930s for the treatment of pneumonia, and penicillin became available after 1941. Blood transfusion techniques were perfected, particularly during the war. X-ray technology developed, and the scope of medical investigation was widened. Just as these new technical advances occurred, the ad hoc system of medical services cobbled together after the First World War reached crisis-point.

The crisis focused on the hospitals. The voluntary hospitals, founded by charities, had increased the number of available beds by 33% between 1929 and 1938, increasing staff numbers in a similar way. To finance this expansion they had shifted from using voluntary contributions as their main source of income to schemes based on pre-paid contributions; 400 contributory schemes extended the idea of pre-payments to hospital medicine, and generated the demand for hospital care, as of right. Yet despite this financial boost, by 1937 three out of ten voluntary hospitals faced deficits. Clearly a new system of funding was required. Equally some kind of centralisation would be demanded, particularly if public funds were to be deployed in the hospital sector. The Poor Law had been abolished, finally, in 1929, but the old Poor Law hospitals had mostly survived, and only a minority had been transferred to municipal control. The scene was set for a new reform with three premises; a right to medical services, including specialist and technical services; a coordinated system of hospitals, with comparable standards; and the use of public funds to maintain the hospital network.

The protagonists for the reform were the trade union movement and the Labour Party, recovering from the disasters of 1926, Ramsey McDonald and the great depression. This time, the advocates of cautious change were the Conservatives who realised that Labour must be given its due, just as the Liberals had in 1911. Like the medical profession, the Conservatives produced their own blueprint for a National Health Service, but really sought only to extend National Health Insurance whilst retaining as large a private sector as possible. Predictably the British Medical Association endorsed this, seeing the general practitioners at the centre of a new health service and their fee-paying patients as the guarantees of quality. The Second World War tipped the balance against cautious reform. Once again, the working population wanted a return for its commitments to the war. The Emergency Medical Service, organised to coordinate the hospital sector for war-time purposes, increased the number of hospitals beds available by 50% and injected the necessary technology, money, and planning. When the Labour Party won the general election of 1945, its opponents feared that it would establish a state medical service. General practitioners working for salaries from health centres would constitute the first line of this new service, with general and specialist hospitals in a coordinated network acting .. as a reserve. The propaganda of the Conservative Party and the British Medical Association (BMA) was directed against this prospect, as if it were real. Labour's supporters saw their government introduce a Bill for a National Health Service in 1946, and enact it in 1948. This was to be 'a jewel in Labour's crown', the greatest public institution in the new socialist Britain.

Unfortunately, the reality did not conform to either fantasy.

The political pressures for a comprehensive, state-run National Health Service were so great during the Second World War that even the Conservative Party and the BMA produced blueprints for such a service. For a time the reformers were in the ascendant, and were able to ensure that change occurred. They failed, however, to agree on the objectives of their reform. The Beveridge Report of 1942 is traditionally taken as the foundation of the NHS. That report was the main element in the war-time planning for peace-time reconstruction. The war-time coalition government had to submit to pressure for social reform during this war, just as in the First World War. The war had to be worth fighting, and therefore the poverty and misery of the depression years had to be counteracted by government initiative. Almost inevitably the reconstruction programme was dominated by reformers, who were able to pick up the arguments for reform that had been developing before the war began. Perhaps the most potent of these arguments came from a curious alliance between the TUC and the British Medical Association. The alliance had developed ostensibly around the isue of industrial injury compensation, but grew into a concerted demand for a new system of sickness benefit and industrial injury compensation, and also for reconstruction of the nation's medical services.

The TUC and the BMA in Alliance

The TUC had been involved in a long-standing conflict with the commercial insurance companies that administered the National Health Insurance and industrial injury compensation. For commercial reasons the insurance companies did not like paying large sums of money if they could avoid it. In cases of industrial injury they encourage the claimants to opt for lump-sum payments following injury, rather than long-term benefits. In general, workers preferred the lump-sum payments, which seemed to represent money lost through injury, and did not think about future wages forfeited through disability, until it was too late. The TUC also resented the influence that insurance companies had over NHI, and their enthusiasm for minimising sickness benefit payments. Over a period of more than a decade the TUC had developed the demand for 'neutral' control of benefit payments.

The other partner in the alliance, the BMA, joined the TUC because it was under pressure from reforming voices within the profession. The Medical Practitioners' Union (MPU) was growing and agitating for better conditions in general practice. The Socialist Medical Association (SMA) had increasing influence in municipal services, particularly in the London Country Council area, and was actively involved in improving municipal hospitals and clinics. This presented a challenge to the BMA's argument that medical autonomy from local government control was all-important for good quality medical care. And the general poor health of the working population was being converted from a professional into a public and political issue. The BMA therefore had little option but to go with the tide. Cooperation between the BMA and the TUC developed throughout the 1930s, despite medical misgivings about the trade union movement and trade unionists' attacks upon the poor quality of general practice. Cooperation turned into coordinated action at the time of the Royal Commission on Workmen's Compensation in 1938. This brought the issues of insurance company control of benefits, and the quality of industrial health service care to a head. The employers made the mistake of boycotting the Royal Commission and so damaged their reputation that private industry, and the Conservative Party, were unable to exert a negative influence on the Beveridge Report.

The BMA-TUC alliance was to continue after Beveridge. When the post-war Labour government began working on the proposal for a comprehensive, state-run medical service, it had to reconcile two conflicting viewpoints within its own ranks. The left of the labour movement, represented by the Socialist Medical Association, envisaged a health service very different from that anticipated by the TUC, in its alliance with the BMA. The SMA wanted a service that was, in effect, an extension of its own power-base, in the municipal hospitals and clinics. The SMA was hostile to the voluntary hospitals, run by charities, and to private medicine in general. Its objectives were not only to provide a free medical service for the whole population, but for the service to be based upon health centres used by general practitioners employed on a salaried basis by local government. The voluntary and private hospitals were to be taken over, but also handed over to local government as a further contribution to the municipal hospital network.

The TUC, on the other hand, had a much narrower interest in a National Health Service. First of all, it wanted to obtain specialist medical attention for the working population. Part of its concern arose because a proportion of the working class had become accustomed to pre-paid medical care at specialist level, through the contributory schemes. The TUC also needed to establish centres of treatment for industrial injuries and disease, and sources of adjudication in compensation cases. (The famous Manor House Hospital in London was established by the TUC for these purposes). The trade unions also needed the support and services of general practitioners to provide an industrial health service independent of management control. They were therefore concerned about improving the quality and quantity of general practice medicine. These concerns had been the basis for TUC approaches to the BMA during the pre-war period, promoted by Labour notables like Ernest Bevin.

The British Medical Association was concerned, above all, with the issue of professional power. It was concerned to defend the independence of doctors from the state, and to increase their decision-making powers over medical care at the expense of both commercial insurance companies and local government. It worked to shape the future NHS to achieve these ends, advocating autonomous general practitioners, the retention of private medicine, and opposition to municipal control of health services. However the BMA did accept that government subsidy was needed to rescue the hospital service from bankruptcy and had learned from the experience of the war time Emergency Medical Service that centralised control and improved financing could go hand in hand without prejudicing professional power. The profession's leaders also acknowledged that free medical services should be extended to a larger part of the population, provided that private medicine was not jeopardized. They realised that the TUC with its narrow perspective on health care, could be a useful ally in supporting the demand for improved hospital services without necessarily challenging their demand for professional dominance of those services.

Aneurin Bevan, the left-wing Minister of Health in the Labour government, had to reconcile the two approaches. The concessions which Bevan made to the medical profession have been a source of anger within the trade union movement since then. The British Medical Association had shifted its ground considerably in accepting the idea of a National Health Service, and in associating itself with the TUC. However it was held back by its own conservatism, and its members were unwilling to become salaried civil servants. The balance of power within the profession shifted away from reforming forces, just as reforms became possible. The BMA struck its flag on the issue of professional independence and forced Bevan to reject the ideas of the SMA.

Bevan's success in negotiations with the medical profession lay in his ability to divide the hospital consultants from the general practitioners. He offered the consultants a new hospital system, paid for by the government but under their effective control, in which they could continue with private medicine. The general practitioners, left unsupported by the hospital specialist, had to accept an extended panel system incorporating the whole population. This left little scope for large-scale private medicine, and was certainly not what the GPs really wanted. Nevertheless they reluctantly accepted Bevan's proposals because of the promise of increased security, without the degrading competition for patients that had marred the pre-war panel system. Bevan also gave general practitioners increased influence over their own administration. Nearly 50% of the places on the new Family Practitioner Committees were occupied by professionals, compared with 10% on the earlier Insurance Committees. General practitioners (GPs) were to be independent contractors to the National Health Service, and not made into salaried employees of it.

The SMA lost on all but one of its principles, the extension of free services to the whole population. Health centres were not to be the basic unit of the new health service, general practitioners were not to become salaried employees, and municipal control was rejected in favor of centralised control by a national ministry. Bevan's only concession to the left was to leave local government in control of its system of maternity and child care clinics, and of the School Health Service. When the National Health Service began operation in 1948 it certainly did meet the needs of the nation. Yet it was shaped largely by the medical profession, in the medical profession's interest, and the profession's alliance with the TUC was to be short-lived.

Shaping the NHS in this way, Bevan un
left within his own party. That defeat ha
within the labour movement, and the issu
still generates more anger than the questic
services, despite the fact that private
symptom of a much more pervasive profes

CHAPTER 2

The Lean Decade

The NHS was created just as the post-war Labour government lost its grip on the nation. Labour had been drawn into an alliance with the USA, becoming economically and then politically dependent on an increasingly aggressive American government. The beginnings of the Cold War had swept Labour into anti-Communist campaigns in Korea, Malaysia, Greece and Britain. The Socialist Medical Association, already soundly defeated in the run-up to the NHS Act, became further marginalised because of its substantial Communist membership. The rival attitude, based on the tacic agreement between the BMA and Bevin's faction of the TUC, set the scene for the next 30 years of the NHS. The labour movement dispensed with its 'own' experts – the SMA – and abdicated responsibility for the new health service to a bigger, more powerful cadre of experts – the mainstream of the medical profession.

The post-war economic recovery was slow and uneven. The Retail Price Index rose from 100 in 1947 to 130 in 1950, and devaluation of the pound occurred in 1949-50. Trade union enthusiasm for Labour government wage restraint began to melt towards the end of the decade, with a succession of dock strikes marking the end of the industrial honeymoon, and with the growth within the TUC of a serious challenge to government economic and foreign policy.

The young health service was caught up in the economic problems, and rapidly became a target for Conservative attack. At the time of the Beveridge Report it had been estimated that the future NHS would cost £170 million to run each year. By the time the NHS Act was introduced, in 1946, the estimate had increased slightly to £180 million per year, with less than 70% of this coming from the Exchequer. The actual cost in the first year of the NHS was £402 million, with £305 million contributed by general taxation. The ophthalmic services, expected to cost less than £1 million, checked in at £22 million in that year, a precise measure of the unmet need for optical care. The new dental services, expected to cost £10 million, cost £34 million, another graphic pointer to the huge needs not catered for by the earlier system. The economic misjudgements of the pre-NHS years rebounded on the Health Minister, Aneurin Bevan. Under Tory pressure to economise, he called for reduced spending on drugs, through more 'rational' prescribing by family doctors. Outflanked to his right by the Labour Cabinet, Bevan resigned after the government re-introduced charges for optical and dental services in 1951, taking with him a young hero of the left, Harold Wilson. A Conservative electoral victory later the same year permitted a further rise in health charges, and prompted an SMA petition campaign against them that raised nearly one quarter of a million signatures.

The Conservatives won one political argument about the NHS even before they won the 1951 election. The Labour assumption that the costs of health care might *decrease* as the new NHS made the nation healthier, collapsed as the financial costs of the health service appeared to escalate. On the basis of this early inflation of health care costs, the Conservatives were able to argue that resources were finite, but demand was infinite. The argument has ricocheted down the decades, side by side with Labour's belief that 'experts know best'. From that electoral turn-around, until the end of the decade, Labour could only fight defensive battles for its Welfare State. To its credit, the Labour Party held off the main Conservative attack in the lean decade, the attack on 'wasteful bureaucracy'.

In 1953 the Conservative government opened an enquiry into the costs of the NHS. Efforts were made to placate the Labour opposition, which feared that this was a backdoor way of mutilating the health service. The enquiry, held by the Guillebaud Committee, relied heavily on a study prepared by two academic advocates of the Welfare State, Brian Abel-Smith and Richard Titmuss. The committee's conclusions, published as the Guillabaud Report in 1956, crushed the Conservative attack. Analysing the dramatic increase in government expenditure on the health service, the report showed that the devaluation of sterling was more to blame than unchecked spending. Allowing for the change in the value of money, and for the initial miscalculations, the NHS was found to be very

cost-effective. The *real* net rise in costs between the 1949 and
1954 was only £11 million, although devaluation made it appear
to be £59 million. As a proportion of the Gross National
Product, the net cost had fallen (because the national income
was rising) from 3.75% in 1949-50 to 3.25% in 1953-54. The
population has also increased, so that the cost per head of the
NHS was the same in 1954 as it had been in 1949. For the
moment the Conservative's economic argument – 'finite
resources, infinite demand' – collapsed, and the Tory
government could only shelve, not contradict, Guillebaud's
Report.

   Health policies was now blocked by a left-right stalemate.
Labour had its health service, but had lost control of the
government. The NHS was a compromise between medical and
social interests, with medical interests dominant in key areas like
control and priority-setting. The Conservatives had regained the
government, had a natural association with medical interests,
but could not make progress in changing the overall policy. The
'lean decade' was lean because no substantial change could occur.
Only the trends established with the NHS in 1948, could
evolve, and then only slowly. The 'period of stability' advocated
by the Guillebaud Report persisted throughout the years of
growing prosperity, in the fifties.

Slow Progress

The Conservatives could not dismantle the NHS, but neither did
they intend to overfeed it. Every aspect of the new health service
was altered by Conservative policy, directly or indirectly, acting
alone or in alliance with professional interests. The staffing and
funding of the newly nationalised network of hospitals had to be
worked out. Arguments about their administration had to be
resolved. New mechanisms for agreeing pay levels and terms of
service had to evolve. Both training and service work needed
rationalisation and refinement. And the government had to pay
some attention to ensuring that the NHS really worked to
people's benefit, at least in the parts of the health service where
conditions were scandalous or the consumers publically critical.
These problems were Labour's legacy to Churchill, Eden and
Macmillan, and were approached in Conservative style, with
minimal funding and a stern resistance to any decisive and

determined action that favoured public rather than private interests.

Their tightest grip was on capital spending – the renovation of old buildings and the construction of new ones. The NHS had inherited nearly 3,500 hospitals in Britain. Nearly half of these had been built before 1891, and 1 in 5 before 1861. The Second World War had stopped both renovation and new hospital construction, so that nearly twenty years of physical neglect had accumulated by the turn of the decade. The government's answer was to hold back building programmes. Capital spending on the NHS actually fell from 0.8% to 0.5% of national capital formation between 1949 and 1954. Figure 1 shows how NHS capital spending compared with the running costs throughout the decade. When the political log-jam broke in the 1960s, a new phase of building began, just as the first warnings of economic down-turn appeared.

Figure 1
Hospital Current Spending and Capital Spending as Percentages of Total Spending on Health and Personal Services, 1949-1979

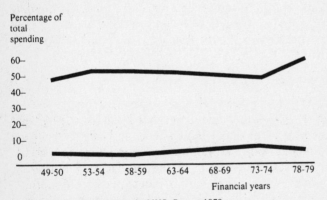

Source: Royal Commission on the NHS. *Report*, 1979.

Community Health Services, particularly general practice, were the second neglected area of capital investment within the NHS. The health service had preserved and intensified the worst features of pre-war general practice by leaving GPs as independent contractors *to* the NHS, rather than making them employees *of* the NHS. The system of paying GPs a fixed sum for each person on their list encouraged inflation of list-size beyond the limits of efficient management. A study of 55 practices in industrial areas of England, carried out just after the NHS was founded, prompted its author to say:

> the working environment of general practitioners in industrial areas was so limiting that their individual capacity counted for very little. In the circumstances prevailing, the most essential qualification for the industrial GP ... is ability as a snap diagnostician − an ability to reach an accurate diagnosis on a minimum of evidence ... the worst elements of general practice are to be found in those places where the greatest and most urgent demand for good medical care ... some conditions of general practice are bad enough to change a good doctor into a bad doctor in a very short time. These very bad conditions are to be found chiefly in industrial areas.
>
> (J.S. Collings, 'General Practice in England today', *Lancet*, 1950).

A review of general practice published in 1965 but describing the level achieved in the 1950s, found wide discrepancies between areas. In working class areas 80% of surgeries were built before 1900, and only 5% had been built since 1945. In middle class areas 25% of surgeries were post-war constructions, and 50% pre-dated 1900. Health centre building mimicked hospital construction. Forty health centres were built in the first twenty years of the NHS.

Growth Despite Restraint

Yet the health service grew, and in its first decade achieved a great deal. The growth came through increased staffing and better deployment of more equipment and more technical expertise. The old Poor Law infirmaries mainly serving working class communities, benefited from the specialists, laboratories and X-ray facilities that they had previously lacked. According to Julian Tudor Hart, 'a huge backlog of gynaecological surgery was shifted in the 1950s, the accumulated discomfort and misery of the neglected pre-war generations of working claass mothers'. A survey of attitudes towards the NHS, at the end of the lean decade, said:

> when thinking of the health service mothers are mainly conscious of the extent to which services have become available in recent years. They were more aware of recent changes in health services than of changes in any other service ... doctors came second to

Figure 2
The Growth of Hospital Staff in England and Wales, 1949-1969

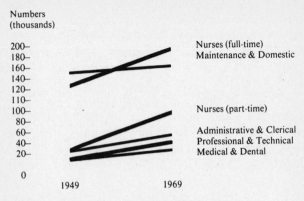

Source: D. Stark-Murray, *A Blueprint for Health*, 1973.

Figure 3
Staffing Changes Within Specialist Medicine, 1949-1956

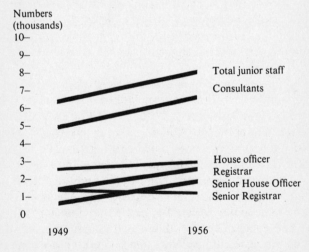

Source: Adrian Tibbit, *The Politics of Medical Manpower*.

relatives and friends in the list of those who have been helpful in times of trouble.

(*Family Needs and Social Services*, Political and Economic Planning, London 1961). The growth in staff was the main

mechanism for redistribution of specialist and technical services.
Figure 2 shows the growth of hospital staff in England and
Wales in the first twenty years of the NHS. Figure 3 illustrates
the change within specialist medicine itself, between 1949 and
1956. New professionals, like the laboratory technicians,
appeared whilst older professions like nursing and
physiotherapy expanded. A hierarchy of medical
'specialists-in-training' grew under the feudal lordship of a
growing body of hospital consultants. As staff numbers
expanded inside elderly hospitals, successive Ministers of Health
had to answer new questions: how should they be organised?
Who is in charge? What should staff be paid? How are they to
be trained?

Controlling Voices

The easiest question to answer was the question of power, of the
choice of controlling voices in the NHS. The new health service
inherited a variety of management styles from pre-1948
hospitals, ranging from local government committees to Boards
of Governors patronised by the charitable and cultured.
Common to almost all styles, however, was a functional
tripartite leadership; the medical director organised medical
care, the matron ran nursing and nurses (both on and off the
wards), and the lay administrator looked after the business end
of hospital care. A report published in 1954, by the Bradbeer
Committee, endorsed this troika, but qualified its collectiveness.
Hospitals could be run by a team of three, said Bradbeer's
Report, but *groups* of hospitals linked together for efficiency
needed one-man management, and that could only come from a
lay administrator. Medical directors and matrons had a
practical, day-to-day administrative role, but no more. Or,
rather, little more. The committee that governed hospitals, and
supervised matrons, lay officers and chief directors alike, could
and should have some medical representation on them. Rarely,
nursing experience would be beneficial to their decision-making,
and occasional room could be made for the exceptional matron.
On no account, however, should other staff be allowed on such
bodies – 'we should deplore any move in the direction of a
syndicalist structure', said the Bradbeer Report.

Pay and Professionalism

Working out how to pay the growing workforce was not so easy as dismissing syndicalist structures. Before 1948, health workers had faced a range of employers, were poorly organised (in trade union terms), and tended to belong to professional groups rather than TUC unions. Organisations like the Mental Hospital and Institutional Workers Union (MHIWU) and the Association of Scientific Workers were to become components of much bigger and more powerful unions (COHSE and ASTMS respectively) later on, but when the NHS was founded they were overshadowed by the Royal College of Nursing (RCN), the Royal College of Midwives, and a range of other specialist professional groups. The coordination of the hospitals into the Emergency Medical Service during the Second World War demanded and permitted better organisation of the chaotic systems of determing staff pay. The wartime Rushcliffe Committee reviewed nursing pay, and involved professional bodies and trade unions as well as local government and hospital management in its work. The Royal Colleges of Nursing and Midwifery dominated staff representation on that committee, and caried on to do so on its successor, the Nurses and Midwives Whitley Council. 'Whitleyism' was born with the NHS, and was the Labour answer to the nightmare of pay negotiation. Nurses and Midwives had a Council, in which their representatives could argue their case with negotiators from the Ministry of Health. Two other Whitley Councils, inspiringly named 'A' and 'B', did the same for health workers dealing directly with the ill, like speech therapists, radiographers and chiropodists, and those with technical functions, like laboratory technicians or hospital engineers. The men from the Ministry could recommend a settlement reached in the Whitley Council to the Government for acceptance or rejection. The Whitley Council system appeared to allow for both multi-party negotiation and government 'independence' from such negotiations. In practice multi-party negotiation fixed and legitimised the expression of staff representation, and the division between professionals and unionists, as much as it reflected the pre-1948 complexities. Government 'independence' was also more a strategy than a solution, for the Health Ministry was always subordinate to its paymaster, the Exchequer, and the Whitley Council merely permitted the government to interfere in pay negotiation without appearing at the table.

Predictably, conflict over pay developed soon after the NHS was founded. In 1948 health workers' unions demanded a wage increase to match that won by local government manual workers. The management side on the Whitley Councils faithfully reflected the Labour government's pay policy, but under pressure allowed for a small wage rise – and blocked further increases for ancillary workers for two years. Nurses' pay negotiations started badly, with a protest over the deduction of national insurance from student nurses' salaries, in 1948. They commenced in earnest in February 1949, dragged on for a year because the management side of the Whitley Council again refused to breach government pay restraint, and ended when the nurses' organisations referred their demand to arbitration. They won, and had their pay increase back-dated.

Recourse to arbitration became a standard technique for health workers' organisations in the fifties. Between 1948 and 1955, 26 of the 53 major settlements in the NHS were the result of arbitration. All but two settlements were referred to arbitration by the staff side of Whitley Council, and 16 of these were 'won' by the health workers. The bulk of these arbitration cases were dealt with by the Industrial Disputes Tribunal (or its predecessor, before 1951, the National Arbitration Tribunal), which became the favoured mechanism for resolving disputes in industries with weak union organisation, or where unions posed no credible strike threat to their employers. Between 1951 and 1959, 105 of the 1,277 awards made by the IDT went to NHS unions, and the NHS ranked third amongst the applicants for arbitration.

Arbitration helped health workers' organisations to overcome their weaknesses, at least in part, but it could not prevent erosion of pay levels (compared with industry and local government) throughout the fifties. The application of government pay policy in the protracted negotiations of Whitley Councils, reinforced by the Conservative principle of underfunding the NHS, made the health service into a low-pay area for the next thirty years, and set off a chain of industrial conflicts. The fifties principle of arbitration, of third-party involvement in settling arguments, also shaped industrial relations inside the NHS well into the eighties, in two apparently contradictory ways. The right to make a *unilateral* referral to *binding* arbitration was ended in 1959, by the Conservative government, and that removed the main negotiating weapon of health service unions and professional organisations alike. Their only option was to develop industrial muscle, and this they did in the sixties and seventies. Even so, nostalgia for the strike-free days of third-party arbitration survived, particularly in the professional bodies. In the seventies these came to envy and emulate the medical profession, which had also learned the value of arbitration in the fifties, but in a different way.

The Review Body System

From the beginning of the National Health Service, the doctors were a special case. That is hardly surprising, for they were architects and co-beneficiaries of the NHS, had enormous political significance for Labour, and in a sense were the key workers in the new health service. Unlike other health workers, they could represent themselves through simple, straightforward mechanisms almost completely controlled by a single body, the British Medical Association. Unlike other health workers, they retained their presence in an alternative health care system, the shrunken but still real sector of private practice, which offered at least the dream of security if life inside the NHS became intolerable. Equipped with a relatively simple negotiating machine, and able to withdraw from the NHS (in theory at least) without withdrawing from medicine itself, the profession could have become both militant and direct in its demand for higher incomes. Apart from a brief period in the fifties, it did neither. Instead doctors opted for a strange but attractive blend of 'Whitleyism' and third-party arbitration. They did so because the profession was united in its representation, but divided in its relationships with the NHS.

The complex financial relationship established between the NHS on one hand, and the differing interest-groups of doctors on the other, grew out of the wartime Emergency Medical Service, alongside 'Whitleyism'. In 1944 it was decided, by the Spens Committee, that doctors' earnings in the future should take as their baseline medical incomes in 1939. The year was chosen carefully and deliberately. During the war years medical incomes had fallen, and 1939 represented the peak of pre-war earnings. In 1948 the BMA demanded a modest 100% rise on top of the 1939 level, was offered 60% by the Ministry of Health, and began the prolonged negotiation so typical of the NHS. The dispute was settled through arbitration by Dankworts of the High Court, in 1951. He found in favour of the doctors, just in time for a newly elected Conservative government to show its appreciation for its natural allies, by accepting Dankworts' ruling.

For most health workers in the fifties, arbitration over pay was the only way to defeat the hostile government. For the BMA it was a tactic for defeating a Labour government, but not necessarily a Conservative one. The medical profession realised that the 1951 Tory election victory had changed the political climate inside the NHS, but it did not recognise the limits of that change, nor quickly understand where it stood in the lean decade. In 1956 the BMA approached the Health Ministry directly, demanding a 24% pay increase, and was rebuffed. Both the profession and the government then faced a political dilemma. Should the doctors attack *this* government in the same way that they had fought with Labour? If they did, and won, what effect would that have, in the year of Suez? Should the government treat the medical profession, its main allies inside the NHS, in the same way that it tried to treat other health service workers, by holding their incomes down? Would that tactic promote medical militancy, damage the National Health Service in the year of the Guillebaud Report, and give Labour another weapon against the Conservative Party?

The dilemma was resolved by a stock remedy – a Royal Commission on ways of determining doctors' pay. The BMA understandably saw this as a diversion from direct settlement of its claim, and threatened to organise the withdrawal of doctors from the National Health Service. Its militancy was sabotaged by the defection to the government viewpoint of the chairman of the BMA's own negotiating committee, Sir Russel Brain! As President of the Royal College of Physicians he was effectively chief consultant as well as chief negotiator, and wisely put the consultants' interests in the NHS in front of the BMA's interests in industrial action. He realised that fellow consultants were not going to jeopardise their privileged (and improving) position in a growing health service, to join in a campaign that was to be determined by the willingness of independent – contractor GPs to withdraw from their contracts with the NHS. The BMA was crippled, just as it had been in the run-up to the foundations of the NHS, when Bevan divided the profession and bought the co-operation of the consultants against the general practitioners. This time a Conservative government used Bevan's tactic, in defence of a health service their political enemies had created eight years previously. Both the Tory government and the medical profession had become prisoners of Labour policies that they once had hoped to influence and modify. If the National Health Service was a compromise that benefited capital and professional interests as much as it benefited the working population, it also restricted those interests by making them accommodate to people's needs. The 1956 doctors' pay dispute was one of many examples of how capital, the state, the small traders of professionalism, and the working class historically determined each other's expression in the complex power struggles within the Welfare State.

Professionalism Versus Solidarity

Why was the BMA sabotaged by the defection of one man, or one group of members? Why did not the general practitioners carry on their campaign, independently of the consultants, and withdraw from the NHS? A decade later, they tried with a similar pay claim, but in 1956 the pecking order of medicine kept general practitioners in the lowly place, and they genuinely feared extinction. Progress in medicine was occurring in the hospitals, and was controlled by the consultants. Many general practitioners feared that hospital consultants wanted them out of the way, and would welcome the withdrawal of GPs from the health service as a useful purge of unnecessary doctors. Sweden and the USA, were to demonstrate that health services (one socialised, the other private enterprise) could be run without general practitioners at all, and British GPs were probably rightly suspicious. The NHS had abolished competition for patients, but it had not eradicated medical rivalry. One general practitioner would withdraw from the NHS, at a BMA command, only if he or she could be sure that his or her 'colleague' down the road did the same. Neither would take such action unless the consultants in the local hospital joined in, and Sir Russel Brain had demonstrated that they would not.

The rivalries were made worse by pay differentials. Hospital consultants had ensured that they earned more than GPs, in a ratio of 3:2. Their salaries could be topped up with special awards for 'merit', distributed by committees of fellow consultants, and paid in three grades. The top grade was designed to *double* the consultant's salary. The general practitioners, on the other hand, had opted to be independent contractors. Their income was worked out on a 'pool' system, in which the intended average net income was multiplied by the number of general practitioners to create a pool of money. Allowances for practice expenses were added to the pool, and notional sums equivalent to income from other sources (like private patients) were withdrawn. The pool was then divided up, according to how many patients the GP served, eligibility for allowances, and assorted claims that GPs made for special payments. The end result was that no one general practitioner had the same pay as another, and that high income depended on having large numbers of patients. Since the labour movement had accepted the principle that the 'experts knew best', no attempt had been made to apply quality controls to GPs' payments. Only quantitative throughput counted in determining salary, so that a dedicated and hard-working doctor providing a high-quality service to a relatively small number of people could earn *less* than an unscrupulous GP providing a minimal standard of service to a much larger population.

The conflicts that this system of payment stimulated amongst general practitioners, and between GPs and hospital consultants, were an effective antidote to the solidarity needed to take and defeat Government pay restraint with outside intervention. In 1951 Mr Justice Dankworts had rescued the BMA – but there was no guarantee that another such saviour could be found again. If the profession wanted to control governments, including Tory ones, it would have to develop solidarity within itself, and that would mean an acceptance by general practitioners of the dominance of state-run health care. In the end, they would have to become salaried employees of the NHS, just like the consultants.

Re-affirming Conservatism

Nobody within the political mainstream of medicine in the fifties could tolerate that idea. The general practitioners themselves had a morbid dread of state service, and had been re-assured by the defeat of the SMA and the Medical Practitioners' Union in the forties. The consultants realised that, whilst the NHS would grow, its resources would be distributed in as miserly a fashion as successive Conservative governments could achieve. If money was rationed, the hospital consultants wanted no competition for it. The Conservative government had no desire to see medical solidarity develop, for two reasons; it wanted to spend as little as possible on the NHS, and it wanted a clear line drawn between 'professionalism' and trade unionism. The Tories knew that, if they permitted the consultants their private practice and allowed them to divide up the merit award cake amongst themselves, these privileged doctors would take care not to expand their membership so much that such sources of income would be 'diluted'. Paying the top few a great deal allowed governments to spend less overall, for the top few would cooperate in minimising the incomes of those below them. Such a pay strategy promoted a professional hierarchy that mimicked the class divisions of the society, and it worked very well. Junior hospital doctors were paid very low incomes for incredibly long hours, well into the sixties, and arguably until their strike action in 1975. Their compensation was to be promotion up the ladder to élite status, but as we shall see, this escalation became as contradictory as upward social movement in society at large. When the situation of junior hospital doctors changed, it did so despite, and not because of, their consultant superiors. What the hospital juniors experienced was to be repeated in nursing in the sixties and seventies, and in the non-professional NHS workforce throughout its first thirty years – the highest echelons either did nothing active to improve the incomes of those below them, or they tacitly collaborated in minimising those incomes.

In general practice, the Conservatives had even more opportunity to apply their economic and philosophical principles. A 12% pay rise awarded to the whole medical profession could be reduced to a 7 or 8% increase for GPs, by skilfull manipulation of the pool system of payments. Since part of the GPs' incomes depended on them claiming payment from the pool, each doctor had to develop and sustain a business-like attitude and commercially sound management methods. The quality of the service provided did not really figure in the analysis, since Conservative thought identifies only one kind of excellence – commercial success. General practitioners in the fifties may have had their ideas modified by work in the wartime military civilian health services, but as a group they had a commercial lineage. It was no hardship for them to retain a shopkeeper mentality, particularly when the sharp edges of competition had been smoothed away by state subsidies. The Ministry of Health felt no pain, either, for it both obtained general practice on the cheap and satisfied the dominant ideology. When 'privatisation' of NHS (and local government) work was promoted by a different kind of Conservative government in the early eighties, it came as a novelty to many in the labour movement yet the health service had depended on contracted-out services in the form of the entire general practitioner system for over thirty years. Had Labour recognised that fact earlier, and made serious efforts to create a salaried sector in general practice, would trade union resistance to privatisation elsewhere in health care have had a better start in the eighties?

The dilemma created by the 1956 doctors' pay demand exposed the contradictions between professionalism and unionism in the NHS, and allowed the Conservatives to re-assert their perspective for health, but it did not allow them to make immediate progress. Their ideal solution must surely have been the pay structure agreed for dentists. Like general practitioners, dentists had accepted independent contractor status in 1948. Unlike GPs, their income came from items of service performed – the number of teeth filled, pulled and replaced. No payment was made for people registered on dentists' lists, for there were no such lists. Deprived of a stable income from a stable population, dentists had to concentrate on the throughput of cases and operate in competition with each other. Every government interested in minimising spending negotiated fees for all items at the lowest price possible. The dentists responded by working longer hours than expected, and doing more dentistry than anticipated. The fees that they actually claimed exceeded the expected claims and put dentists' incomes above general practitioners', when convention required them lower. Faced by such 'rate-busting', the Ministry of Health initiated further 'rate-cutting', by reducing the fee payments on each item of service, and so devalued NHS dentistry for the dentists. The growth of private dentistry at the expense of NHS services originated in the independent contractor status negotiated in 1948, and the 'rate' wars of the fifties. If such a solution could have been tried in medicine as well, the Conservatives would have been able to dismantle much of NHS general practice. Instead, they had to make do with a creative compromise .

The Pilkington Report – A Great Relief!

The Royal Commission on doctors' pay, chaired by Sir Harry Pilkington, reported in 1960. It resolved the dilemma that the BMA and the Conservative government had created, and established a new institution within professional politics – the Review Body. Direct negotiation between the medical profession and the Health Ministry was to go, and with it went any prospect for confrontation, militancy, solidarity or any kind of trade union mentality. Instead the medical profession would present the arguments of all its interested groups to a concerned, but independent body, which would discuss and judge the arguments on their merits. This wise body would not be subject to government control, and would have no power to enforce its conclusions on either the NHS or the doctors. Its review of medical arguments about incomes, and government counter-arguments about financial constraints, would lead to the best possible solution in the circumstances, and would triumph by its moral authority alone. By bringing employers, employees and sub-contractors together, the Review Body acted as a refined form of Whitley Council for medicine, but (in theory) without Whitleyism's susceptibility to government interference. By deciding on the final option, the Review Body was to act as arbiter, but without the binding powers of pre-1959 arbitration, and without voluntary self-referral.

The Review Body was to be a mechanism for settling disputes between friends, a way of incorporating one social group into a wider social alliance without destroying the group's identity or independence. Review Bodies became the bridge of choice between the state and its servants for the groups engaged in social control – medicine, the police, the armed forces. For Conservatism the Review Body became an alternative to the Whitley Councils, and the aggressiveness of Conservatism in the eighties prompted 'non-militant' professional organisations like the RCN to renew their pressure for a Review Body for Nursing. In 1960 the medical profession greeted the Review Body with a great sense of relief. The Review Body removed the prospect of confrontation between doctors and the state, and camouflaged the profession's weaknesses. As the doctors described it, the Review Body lifted them out of the market place. The market they were keen to leave was the one where workers sell their labour power; medicine showed no enthusiasm for leaving that other market place, full of tradesmen's stalls.

Falling off the Ladder

Whilst the medical profession and the government were dancing their way out of a pay confrontation, another problem of professionalism was faced, and solved in a way that required a complete reversal of policy in the next decade. The issue was simple. Through medical eyes, there seemed to be too many doctors. The NHS staff expansion had created teams of hospital doctors, under the command of consultants, with a career ladder aimed at consultant status. The ladders filled up rapidly in the fifties, and then movement up them came to a halt as the consultants at the top stayed in position. Too few new consultant posts were created to employ the rising generation of specialists, partly because of underfunding, but probably because the consultants in post were unenthusiastic about creating new rivals. Retirements and deaths did not free enough existing posts, either, and so solutions had to be found before the career structure collapsed. One response was to encourage doctors to drop off the specialist ladder, into general practice. As a result, a cohort of resentful and disillusioned hospital doctors entered general practice seeing it as far from their first choice of work, and bringing to it reduced enthusiasm and the narrower perspectives of hospital medicine. Perhaps the formation of a College (later graced by Royal Status) of General Practitioners in 1952 reflected the GPs' early anxiety about this influx of refugees from the hospitals. The academics in general practice began to assert that they were specialists in their own right. As we shall see, the content of their special skills was to be decided after the specialist status had been achieved, not before.

Those that did not drop of the ladder had to mark time on whatever rung they had reached. Contract changes extended the occupancy of those grades closest to consultant status, but nearer the ground the newly-qualified doctors still clambered onto the bottom of the career ladder. The next step was to turn off this supply of inexperienced staff ambitious for consultantships. This was done by the Willink Report of 1957, which conventional wisdom describes as a classic miscalculation. The Report worked out the requirements for doctors in the future, and proposed a reduction in the numbers of students allowed into medical schools. Willink's committee underestimated the numbers of doctors who formed part of the 'brain-drain' by emigrating (to the USA, Australia and Canada) and also the extra medical staff needed for the new technology being introduced into medicine. It created a real crisis of under-staffing in the sixties, in solving the alleged problem of over-staffing in the fifties, and thereby encouraged the immigration of doctors (particularly from the Indian subcontinent) to fill the unpopular jobs in the NHS.

It is possible to accept that there was a problem of medical over-staffing in the fifties, and that Willink's Report was simply mistaken in its judgements and proposals, but it is not easy. The staffing crisis that prompted Willink's 'error' was due to a blockage in the medical career structure at consultant level. The real issue was whether more consultant posts were *needed* by the health service, but the political issue became one of possibility – was it possible to expand this top grade? Neither a government keen to spend the minimum on public services nor consultants anxious about diluting their power, resources and private earnings, could see much possibility, and therefore much need, to do so. The subsequent expansion of the consultant grade, in the sixties and seventies, demonstrated that the pressure to create posts had been present, but not expressed, only a few years previously. The changes that occurred between these two phases were changes in government philosophy and political administration rather than in medical technology.

Was Willink mistaken? It is not necessary to be a Freudian to be suspicious about apparently simple, innocent errors. In 1958 the Royal College of Surgeons, giving evidence to the Pilkington Committee about entry to medical training, said:

There has always been a nucleus in medical schools of students from cultured homes ... This nucleus has been responsible for the continued high social prestige of the profession as a whole and for the maintainance of medicine as a learned profession. Medicine would lose immeasurably if the proportion of such students were to be reduced in favour of the precocious children who qualify for subsidies from Local Authorities and the state purely on examination results.

For the eminent surgeons, and their eminent colleagues in other disciplines, medicine was a narrow profession neatly slotted into the class culture of Conservatism. It could expand, but only if it needed to, and not because outside interests wanted such expansion. The Willink Committee's sums were not wrong (at the time), simply accurate reflections of medical power and influence over the NHS.

The NHS Shapes Nursing

Medical power shaped the NHS in the fifties, but the NHS shaped nursing. The hospitals were nationalised without the government knowing exactly what it was taking over, and nursing was one aspect of the new health service that was unknown territory to the Ministry of Health. How many nurses were there, where were they, how much training had they had, what was the quality of their training, and how should they be deployed? Just before the foundation of the NHS, a government working party investigated nursing, and described their findings in 1947, in the Wood Report. The working party started from the astonishing wastage rate in nurse education – 54% of entrants to schools of nursing failed to complete their training. The Wood Report blamed oppressive discipline, poor food and low pay as the main causes for this attrition, and criticised poor selection of applicants and inadequate training as well. Discipline, both in ward work and in the nurses' homes, was described as originating from convent life, with attitudes of insularity and self-denial imposed by a psychologically disadvantaged older generation on younger recruits to nursing. Hours of work were long, domestic chores were part of so-called training, food was inadequate in quality and quantity, and recreational facilities were minimal. The Wood Report recognised that exhortation aimed at the Schools of Nursing, by the Health Ministry, was of little value. Structural change in the organisation and staffing of training schools was needed, and the

Report called for real student status for student nurses, selection of senior teaching staff who possessed the 'capacity for developing satisfactory human relationships', improvements in diet and accommodation, normal working hours (based on a three-shift day), and a shorter training course.

The Wood Report was a devastating criticism of nursing, and provoked an angry response from Matrons and nurse tutors. A second investigation of nursing, carried out between 1949 and 1950 by the Nuffield Provincial Hospitals Trust, provoked them again when its findings were publicised. Student nurses made up 60% of ward staff, and spent three quarters of their time working in the wards, rather than in organised tuition. Ward sisters, on the other hand, spent half of their time on ward organisation rather than on patient care, and gave an average of 5 minutes' tuition per day to their students. Wards were generally understaffed, with one sister and one staff nurse per ward regardless of the ward's size. The patients' day began at 5am (or earlier, in some cases), because it took so long for short-staffed nursing teams to prepare wards and patients for the doctors' ward rounds at 9am. The rest of the day was equally stretched out, leaving little opportunity for ill people to rest until lights out at 10pm.

Neither the Wood Report nor the NPHT survey changed nursing in any immediate way, but eventually they initiated lasting changes, despite fierce opposition from senior nursing staff. The 1949 Nurses Act largely ignored the Wood Report, and made only minor changes to nurse education. Schools of nursing remained based on individual hospitals and it was not until 1962 that a minimum size (300 beds) was required of any hospital with an attached school of nursing. The NPHT survey prompted the RCN to mount its own study of nursing, and not surprisingly its results were more favourable to the profession. Nursing then seemed as powerful in opposing change as did the BMA, but the underlying differences between medicine and nursing undermined professional resistance over the following decades. Nursing, unlike medicine, had had its internal problems examined in public. The content of nursing was scrutinised in a way that medicine was to experience in the seventies, but not before. Administrative pressure, trade union action and the work of forward-looking professionals could combine to reform nursing precisely because contentious issues had become public property. No such change occurred in medicine, which continued to demonstrate its collective power to change the NHS rather than be changed by it.

The Reform of Nursing

The changes that occurred on hospital wards and in nursing school adapted nursing to the needs of the NHS. The organisation of nursing work was improved, with experiments in ward size, and in 'team nursing', in which a group of nurses of mixed experience would work together for small numbers of patients on a hospital ward. Efficient organisation emphasised the importance of ward administration. The objective of nurse training was not yet the administrative apparatus created in the late sixties, but the separation of trained nurses from patient care began in the fifties. The education of student nurses, and their slow extraction from routine ward work, also became themes of the fifties reforms. Educational specialists free from ward responsibilities appeared in nursing in the sixties as a response to the pressure for improved training. Domestic work, and more basic tasks in nursing, were shifted to a growing workforce of nursing assistants and nursing auxiliaries. State Enrolled Nurses, originally confined to jobs in mental illness hospitals, with a shorter training than their State Registered Nurse equivalents, were allowed to work in general hospitals to fill the gaps.

The expansion in nursing numbers, and later improvements in nurse training, could occur because staff with less skills and lower wages were recruited from the fifties onwards. The idea that student nurse numbers should be increased, and that these nurses should have genuine student status instead of being cheap labour, was dismissed because of its financial implications. Even cheaper labour was available, and a massive expansion of nurse training could be avoided by a more 'rational' division of tasks within nursing. Such rationality was the product of professional self-interest and the underfinancing of the NHS, and nursing evolved around what was possible rather than what was desirable. The foundation of the NHS made possible developments already inherent in medicine, but in nursing the new health service forced changes on an unwilling profession.

What about the Customers?

What happened to the millions of people who passed through the waiting rooms, wards and pharmacies of the new health service? Where do they fit in the politics of health, during the lean decade?

At the end of the story, and at the end of this chapter! The NHS offered a new service, and the role of the people was to *use* it. The punishing 17 hour day in hospital wards was the price to be paid for access to free services and to medical technology. The long wait in dreary waiting rooms for free GP attention or dental care for all the family was better than the cost of paying for services before 1948. Criticism, or even concern at, the quality of care took second place to more serious work, and a 'consumer consciousness' did not appear, in any organised way until the sixties.

That did not mean that the health service was indifferent to public expectations. People's needs had made the NHS necessary, and continued to influence priorities within it particularly in two aspects of medicine: child-birth and childcare, and mental illness.

Maternity services, and medical facilities for children, were traditional campaigning issues in the labour movement. The alliance of women and labour had created the Ministry of Health in 1919, in an attempt to unify services, and had gone on to promote midwifery, child health clinics and family planning services throughout the inter-war period. In the fifties this pressure for improvements in services continued, and was concentrated on the place of birth, the prevention of infectious disease in children, and the use of hospitals by children.

The Place of Birth

In the fifties women had their babies at home, in maternity units by midwives and GPs, or in hospital labour wards. Their antenatal care was provided in GPs' surgeries, or at a local authority clinic run by local authority midwives, or in an antenatal clinic attached to a local hospital. The place of birth was chosen according to the availability of services rather than the needs (let alone the wishes) of the pregnant woman. The place could be changed during labour if complications developed. A woman expecting to deliver her baby at home might haemorrhage, or become exhausted by a long labour, or show signs of blood-poisoning, and be transferred to the local hospital. In 1958 one third of babies were born at home, one fifth in GP maternity units and nearly half in hospitals. The greatest problem for the health service was not the complexity of its maternity care, but its failure to match the women with the best possible place of birth. The hospital labour wards concentrated obstetric and midwifery skills, alongside blood transfusion facilities and operational theatres, and were the obvious place for women with complicated pregnancies. Maternity units run by GPs, and confinements at home, were suitable for women with uncomplicated pregnancies. Antibiotics were available to treat postnatal infections, community midwives and GPs were skilled at obstetrics (simply through practice), and 'flying squads' could bring expert help, anaesthetics and blood transfusion equipment from hospitals to maternity clinic or maternal home should an otherwise entirely normal pregnancy go wrong at the last moment. In practice, this neat division broke down.

Modern obstetricians like to say that pregnancies can only be described as uncomplicated retrospectively − when the mother has delivered her child in the safety of a modern hospital labour ward. During the 1950s women with complicated pregnancies, women in ill-health before and during pregnancy, and women who had problems with previous pregnancies, were encouraged to have their babies at home, or in a GP maternity unit, rather than in the safety of the hospital labour ward. Sometimes this encouragement came from midwives and GPs, who misjudged risks. Sometimes the women themselves refused to consider a hospital birth, despite the risks they ran. Often the encouragement came from hospitals with more pregnant women booked in than beds available. The result was a disaster. Women allocated to give birth at home attended antenatal care less often than women booked for hospitals confinement, had complications diagnosed at a later stage, and had less follow-up if complications developed. Probably one in three of such women did develop complications that threatened the pregnancy, and many were transferred to hospital maternity departments before the onset of labour, or during labour itself. They were much more likely to die in or after labour, or to lose their babies, than women who had experienced appropriate and adequate antenatal care, and who had access to a suitable safe place of birth. Every fourth pregnancy seemed safe enough for a home confinement, and the technical problem lay in choosing the right one and persuading the others that home births were not for them. The political and economic problems, however, were very different, and solving them took precedence.

When this situation was exposed by the investigations of the Cranbrook Committee, between 1956 and 1959, the solution seemed relatively simple. Specialist services should be expanded to meet the needs of those women who, on balance, would be running 'excessive' risks by delivering their babies too far from the skills of hospital obstetricians. The Cranbrook Committee thought that 30% of pregnancies could safely end as home births, once the midwives and doctors refined their selection criteria. The target for 'institutional confinement' would therefore be 70% of all births.

For once, a recommendation was rapidly implemented. By 1965 the Cranbrook target had been reached, and by the late seventies home confinements were the pursuit of the eccentric. This unusually rapid change occurred as part of the general expansion of hospitals at the expense of community services, and its speed reflected the enthusiasm of hospital obstetricians for complete control of maternity care. The first step was to increase the number of births in GP maternity units (which were cheaper to run than hospitals) whilst reducing the control the GPs had in those units. The second step was to reduce the postnatal stay in maternity units so that more women and their babies could pass through labour wards. Once increased efficiency and falling birth rates had combined to ease traffic-flow problems in hospital maternity wards, the GP maternity units could be dispensed with. As usual, the cult of expertise over-ruled all other considerations. Maternity care might mimic a cattle market, but that was the price of safety.

Children in Hospital

Doctors were not the only ones who 'knew best'. Nurses had strong feelings about how hospitals should run, particularly when it came to looking after ill children. Children admitted to hospital in the fifties were sometimes put into adult wards, with little or no separation from the sights and sounds of ill and perhaps dying adults. Their stay, even if in a special ward for children, tended to be prolonged, with infrequent and rigidly controlled visits. Minimal contact with parents was thought to be 'good', particularly amongst nursing staff, because it reduced emotional outbursts from frightened, lonely toddlers and small children confined to beds in dull and unfamiliar wards. Their medical treatment itself was questionable, particularly with commonplace operations like tonsillectomy. About 200,000 children had their tonsils removed each year, and by the late fifties nearly one in three children had undergone tonsillectomy before the age of thirteen. The objective of all this surgery (which was not without risk) was to reduce the frequency of throat and ear infections, but close study of countries with low rates of operation (like Sweden) showed that the operation made no difference. Throat and ear infections continued to plague some chidlren, despite their curative surgery, and all the surgical skill, post operative pain and occasional deaths from haemorrhage, were wasted.

The kinds of treatment experienced by children, and their parents, in the new health service, gave rise to the first real campaigns to improve the NHS and make it sensitive to popular feeling. The Platt Report of 1959 recognised the harsh world of children's wards in hospitals, and advocated open access for parents and a more child-like environment. A prolonged war to implement the Platt Report followed in the sixties, with every hospital a battle-ground. It has not become a political issue, or even a political landmark, probably because the war was eventually won, yet the transformation of paediatric medicine that began in the fifties depended on the active response of parents to intolerable conditions, and was one of the first triumphs of progressive reformers after 1948.

Education for Health

A second triumph was the growth of health visiting as a profession. Before 1948 health visitors had been either local authority employees or voluntary workers recruited by charities working as subcontractors to local government. Their work was mostly with babies and small children, although some worked as contact-tracers for tuberculosis and venereal disease. The foundation of the NHS changed all that. Qualifications became obligatory, and the contracted-out voluntary services disappeared or restricted themselves to local government work with the elderly. The NHS health visitors began to extend their role, to advise on the care of the ill, support of the elderly infirm, prevention of the spread of infection, and to bring a link between the public and specialist services. A survey of the scope of health visiting (The Jameson Report, 1957) described a new kind of health worker, in contact with whole families and communities, taking on problems of mental health and of the care of those discharged from hospital, as well as their existing tasks. With no in-depth casework, and no specialisation, health visitors would become the front-line of the NHS. Their numbers would nearly double in ten years, as would numbers in training.

In reality, health visiting has not flourished as much as the Jameson Report hoped, and it has not become the front-line of the health service, but remains a specialist element within community services. Growth in numbers has not been so spectacular, either, but is has occurred. The success of health visiting lies in its survival as an important component of basic health care, a part of the NHS close to people's lives and concerned with the maintenance of health, not its salvage. The mass vaccination and immunisation programmes that began in the forties and fifties were the basis for the health visitors' preventive approach, and the fruit of it. We no longer see children with polio, diphtheria or smallpox; tetanus is rare, and even whooping cough is less common and less devastating than it was. Preventive medicine worked well, in the early years of the NHS, and created a type of health worker who may become crucial for the renewal of the health service in the future.

Mental Health Care

A third triumph in the lean decade occurred in mental health care. If the children's wards were harsh, and general hospital routine punitive, the mental illness and mental handicap hospitals were scandalously bad. Overcrowded and understaffed, situated in decaying Poor Law Asylums, with minimal funding for essentials like food and laundry, these institutions constrained the mentally ill and handicapped physically out of sight of the general population. Yet their conditions were well known, and the scandal was public.

A parliamentary debate in 1954 had Kenneth Robinson, later a modernising Health Minister in a Tory administration, listing the material shortcomings of these institutions: unsuitable buildings in the wrong places; too few beds; too few staff; too little money. By 1957 an investigative committee had identified ways of improving the asylums, and mental health care generally (the Percy Report), and by 1959 a Mental Health Act had been passed.

This Act did not solve the problems of the asylums, and may even have made the case of the mentally ill more complex in some ways, but it achieved one immensely important, positive change. For the first time 'patients' rights' appeared in a standardised, legal form. Mental illness (and handicap) were redefined, and individual rights clarified, to make compulsory admission to mental hospital more difficult and 'informal' (non-compulsory) admission easier. The service became one available to help the ill, as well as to contain those endangering themselves or the public. Progress in establishing patients' rights may have halted after the 1959 Act, but in mental illness and handicap the breakthrough had finally occurred. The 1959 Act completed the changes in *accessibility* of services started in 1948.

Patients' rights were not enough to restructure mental health care entirely. The asylums became a source of public scandals for the next thirty years, and were consistently underfunded, even by the miserly standards of the NHS. The 1959 Act projected the idea of 'community care' for the mentally ill and handicapped, but devolved statutory responsibility for community services onto local government, not the NHS. In effect, when the health service was obliged to improve its services, it passed the buck. All the residential homes for the mentally handicapped had been transferred from local government to the NHS in 1948. In 1959 the NHS returned the responsibility, but not the buildings. Local government had to rebuild its services, from scratch, under statutory obligation, and progress was slow. Once more, the medical priorities of the National Health Service asserted themselves. Hospitals? Yes, but hospitals for physicians and surgeons first, and people's needs second.

The Lean Decade

The fifties were thin years for change in health care, yet were fat with paradoxes. A skilled workforce was recruited to run new machinery, and new processes, in old plants. The decade began with a shortage of doctors, and the enrolment of 3,000 medically-qualified European refugees. It ended with the threat of excessive medical staff, and an unrealistic reduction in medical school intakes. Yet the unskilled jobs in the NHS were empty because of the domestic shortage and low wages, and were filled by immigration of workers. The lean years began with the Labour government re-instating charges to patients, having abolished financial barriers to medical care only three years previously. And they ended with the Conservatives inheriting an under-funding problem of their own making, and preparing a hospital building programme for the sixties. Patients gained legal rights under a progressive Mental Health Act, but the asylums continued to crumble. Local government regained control of mental handicap services, but local government midwives slowly lost control of maternity care. Doctors surrendered their militancy, with relief, whilst other health workers struggled for confidence, strength and industrial power. So much could have changed, so little did. When the political climate altered in favour of change, the opportunities were fewer and the options narrower. By 1960, the politics of health had set in a pattern that was to last for another twenty years.

CHAPTER 3

Effectiveness and Efficiency?

By the beginning of the sixties, Britain had never had it so good. The post-war boom made classlessness and the end of ideology imminent, if only for those who needed to see such miracles. People seemed better fed, better housed, better educated and better paid than the generation of the 'hungry thirties' had expected, and some sort of social revolution was assumed to be underway.

In health care, this 'revolution' showed itself in all its glory. In the previous decade effective medicines had multiplied at an unparalleled rate. Antibiotics had become everyday 'cure-alls', and the first experiments in oral contraception at last promised easy, full, fertility control. The sixties were the years of the Pill, and family planning began to change from a fringe issue in medicine into a major theme in health care. They were also the years of Thalidomide, the years when the drug industry's unscrupulous pursuit of profit became a public issue.

Machines appeared as the solutions to problems, the essential adjuncts to medical skill. Machines that traced heart rates and rhythms, machines that analysed blood, machines that tracked radioactive chemicals in body organs, machines that measured uterine contractions, all pulsing and whirring and printing out the scientific truths of modern medicine. The isotope scanners, the obstetric monitors, and the cathode tubes of the new coronary care units became the cutting edge of health care, and the essential backdrop to the dramas of birth, illness and death.

These were all the signs of modernisation, the renewal of British industry and social life that was made both possible and essential by the post-war boom. Effectiveness and efficiency became watch-words in industries and organisations showing neither quality, the National Health Service among them. The deployment of new technology became both the problem and the solution for industry, and for health care. New plant and machinery was essential, but who could pay for it, who would run it, and where would it come from in the first place? Both Conservative and Labour governments faced these questions, and each tried to answer them. The Conservatives initiated change (in the NHS at least) but were too closely identified with the restrictive policies of the previous decade to be seen as innovators. Labour took over in 1964, without diverging excessively from Conservatism on issues that were to have enormous impact on the health service, and on politics generally, well into the eighties. Pay restraint became indirect, through incomes policies, rather than direct, through government action. The distribution of power was left unchanged, but its mechanisms were transformed by the incorporation of pressure groups into complex, consensus-management structures. Profit-seeking industries, producing pharmaceuticals and medical equipment, were accepted as normal and necessary suppliers to the state's health service.

In the NHS these modernising trends produced a package of changes that are still represented as individual items, despite their common stock. A qualitative change occurred in the growth pattern of the health service, with a planned hospital building programme that outran itself, and a parallel but unplanned surge in health centre building. The problem of the low pay of so many health workers was 'solved' by changing industrial relations, in favour of incentive and productivity-related payment and better mangement methods. Professional powers were re-organised, with the upgrading of nursing and the incorporation of medicine into an increasingly centralised administration. And consumer pressure blossomed as the growing NHS provided scope for more and more professional responses to people's problems.

New Hospitals, at Last!

The hospitals inherited in 1948 were in urgent need of renovation or replacement by the end of the fifties. They were the wrong design for the new approaches to medicine, in the wrong places, with crumbling structures. In 1962 the Health Ministry, led by Tory Health Minister Enoch Powell, published the *Hospital Plan for England and Wales*. The plan was based on a comprehensive review, on a regional basis, of the NHS hospital stock. It was the first attempt at national planning of health care resources, and it tried to match methods to facilities. Estimates of the number of hospital beds needed per thousand population became 'bed norms', applicable to all health service Regions. The costs of hospital in-patient care were rising, and the Health Ministry took its cue from Oxford Region, which had demonstrated that the average length of stay in hospital could be markedly reduced without impeding the patient's recovery. The elderly sick, and mentally handicapped and ill people, needing long term care, were seen as groups who could be better looked after in 'the community'. Bed norms were fixed so that a reduction in the number of hospital beds would occur, with closure of small hospitals and centralisation of services in large District General Hospitals (DGHs).

The Hospital Plan provided the slogans for the next 20 years of health politics. Care in the community, centralisation of services and increased productivity (by reduced in-patient stay) became themes shared by governments of both parties. Public resistance to closures, particularly where geography and transport systems favoured small hospitals and reduced access

Figure 4

NHS Capital Expenditure and Hospital Planning, 1949-1978

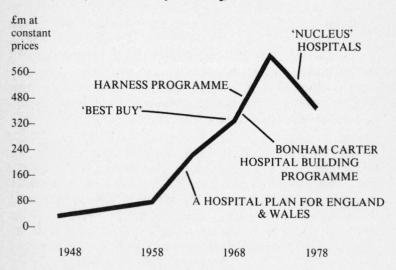

Source: DHSS, *Review of Health Capital*, 1979.

to the centralised DGHs, flared throughout the sixties and seventies. Trade union hostility to closure of large mental illness and mental handicap institutions focused on the implied job-loss, and was only muted by promise of *more* jobs in community care.

Resistance did not impede progress, as defined by the Health Ministry. Figure 4 shows how NHS capital expenditure took off after the Hospital Plan was published.

The building programme was hampered by the preceding decades of neglect. There was no reserve of planning skills in NHS that could keep pace with the money released in the capital programme. Designers borrowed the tower block idea from council housing, promoting large, high-rise slab blocks like the Guy's Tower in London, and Royal Liverpool Teaching Hospital, that were built in single, capital-hungry phases. Alarmed at the costs and complexities of these monstrous buildings, the Department of Health (the Health Ministry's sixties successor) searched for standard designs. First they chose the 'Best Buy' hospitals, built with simple technology to a set pattern, with substantial space-saving and bed norms *below* the levels of the Hospital Plan. Later the DHSS encouraged the 'Harness Programme', based on a flexible standard design that could be assembled in phases and different permutations – a kind of hospital 'Lego'. Taking modernisation to its limits, the Bonham Carter Report (1969) advocated even more centralisation, urging DGHs with 1,000 or more beds to serve populations of up to 300,000, in place of the Hospital Plan's 600-800 bed hospitals for populations of 100-150,000 people.

The rush to centralise could not last. Growing economic problems reduced government enthusiasm for public spending, and the virtues of small hospitals were rediscovered by Keith Joseph, Conservative Health Minister in the Heath government of 1970-74. The last phase of hospital building, the 'Nucleus' hospital programme, aimed to produce modest 300 bed units with the utmost economy in capital and running costs. In theory, these hospitals could be extended when finance permitted. 'Need' had almost vanished from the planning equations, and the end of the sixties boom hinted that another phase of make-shift renovation was imminent.

Can Community Services Catch up?

Community-based health services were no less in need of renovation than the more prestigious hospitals. They were, however, either controlled by local authorities or part of the 'independent contractor' services, and therefore controlled by no-one. The attempts made in the sixties to develop and plan community services demonstrated the advantages of centralised control over local control of services, at least when it came to national planning programmes. It was not simply the unfulfilled expectations of growth, but the variations in attitudes, standards and provision of services, that clinched the argument. Planning just seemed impossible within local authority health services, except at local level, and that could not satisfy the modernising ideology and its society-wide objectives. The document *Health and Welfare: the development of community care* (1963) outlined ambitious plans for growth in community health services and envisaged the coordination of plans for these services in two five-year stretches, from 1962 to 1966, and from 1967 to 1971. *Health and Welfare* noted that variation between authorites was inevitable, and that no common standards of service could be imposed. A staff increase of 39% in health and welfare services was projected for the two five-year plans, with a 42% increase in revenue expenditure and capital spending of £150 million in the first plan and £70 million in the second five-year period. The emphasis, in all this planned growth, was to shift from the provision of particular services to meeting particular needs. Priority client groups were to be mothers with young children, the elderly, the mentally ill and the physically handicapped.

Health and Welfare was ambitious in its hopes for co-ordinated growth, and wrong in several of its predictions. The need for community midwives was overestimated, with 6,500 jobs planned for 1972, despite the growth of hospital obstetrics. In 1971, there were only 4,000 full-time midwives in community services. The need for health visitors was underestimated according to Health Ministry criteria, but even the lower target was not reached. *Health and Welfare* suggested a total of 7,600 health visitors would be at work by 1972, whilst the Department of Health reckoned on 8,600 by 1971. In fact there were only 6,000 employed by 1971.

Similar underestimates retarded growth in the provision of residential places for mentally handicapped adults, and in the constructions of health centres. Health centres were given particularly low priority. Four more were to be added to the 17 already operating in 1963, and another 26 would be planned for the decade. According to *Health and Welfare*, 'the circumstances which now justify their provision do not arise frequently.' Nearly 100 health centres were open by 1970, and 200 more were in the pipeline. The circumstances had arisen more frequently as the rising costs of land and buildings, particularly in urban areas, made general practitioners more interested in capital investment by local authorities. The local authorities themselves saw a chance to incorporate community health services into urban redevelopment, scoring political advantages whilst also tempting doctors anxious about the price of premises. This was planning, of a kind, but it reflected changes in the property market and local ambitions rather than the perspectives of the Department of Health.

General Practice – Half Nationalsied?

General practice was drawn into this modernisation, but well in the wake of the hospital system. With poor facilities, declining morale and unimpressive standards of medical care, general practice was sinking fast. Conscious that general practice could act as a cheap barrier between the population and the attractions of expensive hospital medicine, the DHSS became sensitive to GP fears of extinction by high-technology medicine. The result was the 1966 Family Doctors Charter, promoted by the BMA, but largely borrowed from the progressive Medical Practitioners' Union. The Charter half-nationalised general practice, subsidising premises and support staff for general practitioners, and boosting GP incomes. The General Practitioner's precious 'autonomy' was retained, and no real accountability was demanded in return for so much of the tax-payer's money.

In one sense it was a gain for those seeking the incorporation of general practitioners into the NHS as salaried employees. General practice had demonstrably failed, and needed subsidy to survive. It was not a 'liberal profession', but a claimant on the

Exchequer. The insistence on 'autonomy' was not a reflection of strength, but more a refusal of responsibility. The DHSS was well satisfied with the outcome in 1966, and remains so. Paying all or part of the costs of existing surgeries was (and still is) cheaper than building new ones. Re-imbursing a large proportion of the wages of receptionists, secretaries, managers and practice nurses was preferable to paying the whole bill, especially when general practitioners could be relied on to recruit women workers, at low rates of pay, without encouraging unionisation. Should problems arise with GP services, they could be deflected away from the DHSS, on to the 'autonomous' general practitioners. And should the GPs themselves become difficult, subsidies could be withdrawn and livelihoods threatened.

This approach did more to strengthen the barrier to hospital care than the renewed health centre building programme, and was applied to all the 'independent contractor' health professions – dentists, opticians and pharmacists. Health centres were built at a faster rate, but only for the reasons given, (see Figure 5), and were the selective instrument for improving community services by creating 'centres of excellence'. The bulk of doctors and dentists were excluded from this approach, and

Figure 5
Health Centre Construction, 1948-1980

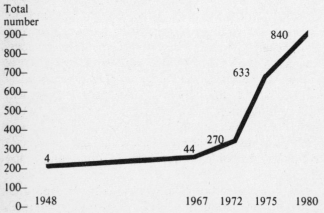

Source: Royal College of General Practitioners, *Trends in General Practice*, 1979.

the NHS concentrated its attention on acquiring the network of nursing, maternal and child health clinics still run by the local authorities.

Low Pay

Before such a takeover could occur, however, the NHS had to be made so efficient that the advantages of central control and planning appeared irresistible. The drive for efficiency demanded that health workers should clarify their roles, and that in turn required a review of their status and income. Professionals were to be incorporated into managerial roles, but only after degrees of professionalism had been established, and a clear demarcation drawn between professional and non-professional workers. The new ranking order of skills was to be marked in the traditional way, by differences of income. The struggle for better living standards was turned into a struggle for efficiency, and professionalism became the dominant component of this efficiency-drive, with productivity in second place.

In the sixties manual workers in the NHS were amongst the lowest paid workers in the country. Men working as porters, or in cleaning or catering departments, were at the bottom of the national pay league; women workers were better paid in relation to other industries, but only because women's pay was so low overall. A quarter of a million health workers were in this manual category, and three-quarters of them were women. Recruitment to jobs had been hampered by the uncompetitive pay rates, and by the sixties the NHS was relying on immigrant labour to fill the lowest-paid, least desirable posts. This largely female, and increasingly black, labour force was poorly paid because the government had no interest in funding the NHS adequately, because of the ample supply of workers (even if only from other, poorer, countries) and because of the low market value of domestic and manual work. Their market status was probably the major obstacle to better pay, even allowing for the relative weakness of health workers' trades unions.

In orthodox terms, the domestic and manual workers were at the bottom of the pile because the essence of health care was contact between patients and skilled professionals. In real terms, the distinction between professional and non-professional workers was not so simple. Contact with patients was potentially greater for non-professionals than for some professional workers. A porter or ward orderly might spend more time with an ill person than did the surgeon who operated on him or her, in the course of an in-patient stay. A nursing auxiliary in a mental illness hospital could easily have more contact with individual patients than did the charge nurse for their ward, and would certainly see more of ill people and do more with them, than the psychiatrist nominally in charge of their care. The differences between professionals and non-professionals were in their special, technical functions rather than in the extent of patient contact. Technical functions like providing comfort and reassurance, help with getting in and out of bed, or a chance to talk, were common enough in the labour market, and were therefore cheap. Operating on duodenal ulcers, interpreting chest X-rays, or reconstructing injured bodies were rarer skills, and commanded a higher price. As we shall see (in Chapter Seven) professionalism is a market concept, not an indicator of patient care.

The market orientation may be unchallengeable in certain circumstances. A motorist badly injured in a car accident needs the surgeon to save life or limbs before the ward nurses can assist recovery, or the ward clerk can inform friends and family. Even then, without the ambulance driver, the blood bank technician and the sterile supplies department, success and survival are not guaranteed, yet the highest paid worker is simply the rarest. Many surgeons work between 60 and 80 hours a week, and the surgeon's reward *could* be a working week of 40 hours, which would allow more surgeons' jobs to be created to meet the unpredictable need for surgery. In the sixties, as now, the surgeons chose financial rewards and took care to restrict their numbers and retain their scarcity-value. Their relatively high incomes, subtracted from the finite resources of the NHS, contributed to the low incomes of their ancillary staff, who were already an expendable workforce drawn from a large reserve of labour. The process of patient care was shaped in the image of the marketplace, and the changes initiated in the sixties reinforced rather than undermined that image.

Productivity and Incentives

The problem of low pay was 'solved' by the open importation of market concepts and management methods. In 1967 the National Board on Prices and Incomes reported on manual workers pay in the NHS. The NBPI was a Labour creation, introduced during the administration of the ex-Bevanite Harold Wilson, as part of the mechanism for imposing pay restraint. It noted the low pay in the NHS, and attributed it to lack of overtime pay, productivity bonuses and incentive payments inside the NHS, compared with other industries. Overstaffing was identified as one cause of this poverty, and the problem was redefined as 'low earning opportunities' rather than low pay. The solutions were stock answers, borrowed from productive industry: productivity deals, work-study specialists, better management, and a 10% bonus in return for a 10% reduction in staffing.

Defining 'productivity' in terms of health care meant defining the contribution of non-professionals to the process of patient care, and was carefully avoided. Overstaffing was assumed to be a problem, since discussion of the idea would expose the market concepts determining the *whole* labour process in the NHS, and upset the professionals keen to retain a reputable, non-commercial image. Work-study was promoted as an answer without too much thought about the objectives of the work – the purpose of the health service, and the roles of those who worked in it. Too much scrutiny of what health workers actually did was avoided, perhaps because past experience (particularly with the investigations of nursing in the forties) had shown it to be contentious. Different groups of health workers could be studied, of course, but the study methods were decided according to the existing distribution of power within the health service. 'Manual' workers in the NHS, like manual workers elsewhere, could be studied by their managers with a managerial perspective. Nurses, who were trying hard to be professionals and escape their manual functions, could also be studied by management, but were pushing hard for assessment to be kept within the profession. Doctors could only be assessed by other doctors, and even that was considered unprofessional!

The alternative to the NBPI's approach was unthinkable. A pay increase that would have given modest relief to the lowest paid amongst NHS staff would have overwhelmed pay differentials. The only solution was to grant an across-the-board increase, keeping differentials intact, and this would have broken the government's pay policy. Any attempt to redefine roles in health care would have upset existing market relationships and have provoked a political crisis. Wilson's government had no desire to 'modernise' the NHS in a way that created political problems for which it was unprepared, or financial demands that could divert money from investment in private industry. Such 'modernisation' as was allowed was designed to streamline a public industry that played a support role in an economy led by the market and in a social structure dominated by Conservatism. 'Modernisation', in health care, involved good, old-fashioned management sense as well as forward planning, and labour market principles as well as twenty-first century technology.

The consequences of the NBPI's advice were not exactly as predicted. Despite efforts to improve NHS management, the introduction of incentive and productivity schemes got off to a slow start. Where productivity deals were negotiated, the relationships between unions and managers began to change. The slow growth in local bargaining at last allowed local unions to play a part in the wages struggle. The end of binding arbitration, in 1959, had deprived health workers of a third-party ally in wage negotiation, and forced their organisations into more aggressive bargaining. Ancillary workers' hourly pay rates matched the rates for equivalent workers in other industries, partly because of this change in their unions, but that had not been enough to improve their incomes overall. Local bargaining, as part of a shift to a more usual industrial status, encouraged local militancy. It was this change, and not simply low pay, that permitted waves of industrial action within the NHS in the seventies. For management, the shift to local bargaining demanded 'responsible' trade unions or professional bodies, and in the seventies trade unionism (of a kind) was to be promoted as a necessary element in NHS management. Nothing could have done more to complicate the management of the health service. Just as all efforts were directed at incorporating professionals (and to some extent, non-professional workers) into a streamlined administration structure, a 'solution' to pay problems created mechanisms for local conflicts that, in themselves, could not end low pay in the health service.

Changing Professionalism

Whilst the productivity of non-professional workers was being questioned, professionalism in health care was also changing. The changes that began in the sixties were designed to exploit new medical technology to the maximum, given restricted NHS budgets and unending, Government-imposed, pay restraint. The workers using the new technology needed coordination, despite their different training and functions, to achieve cost-efficiency. They also needed to learn managerial roles, so that they could be given some responsibility for sharing the resources that the health service used. And they had to be fitted into career-structures that offered promotion from relatively humble and low-paid jobs to higher positions of greater power and improved income, if only because the NHS could not afford to pay all its workers a realistic wage.

The attempts to change professionalism encountered the same obstacles as the hospital building programme. There was a lack of the political skills needed to induce change in resistant interest groups, just as there had been a shortage of architectural experience. And there was too little money, particularly for the salary bill, to make the new structures work as planned.

The administration of the health service was the first to be changed, so that it could become the managerial core of the modernised NHS. Administrative training was rationalised, and a reduction in the length of training was recommended by the Lycett Green Report, in 1963. Annual assessments of NHS administrators, according to Civil Service methods, were also proposed, as were standardised appointment criteria and appointment procedures for managerial posts.

Hospital Consultants were drawn in managerial roles, as much as they permitted themselves to be, following the publication of the first Cogwheel Report in 1967. Produced by a joint working party from the Health Ministry and the Joint Consultants Committee (itself controlled by the BMA), this report proposed new responsibilities for hospital consultants without challenging their power to influence resource allocation. The report advocated that consultants should be grouped into 'divisions' where they would review the services they were providing, arrange to deploy resources efficiently, and cope with management problems as they arose. Cogwheel encouraged the idea of 'operational research', in which research time and money went into evaluating patient care, but opposed the idea of outside scrutiny. The interest that the consultants had in acquiring the local authority clinic system was reflected in the report, which urged further centralisation of the health service. New types of hospital care were discussed, the 'short-stay' and 'overnight' wards, day-care surgery, and 'five day' wards, with the aim of reducing in-patient costs. No suggestions were made that might have challenged the consultants control over a fixed number of beds within their hospital, for Cogwheel was an attempt at partnership between administrative and medical interests, not a warning of a coup.

The dangerous side of modernisation threatened the medical profession a year later, when the Todd Report was published in 1968. This review of medical education, the first since the foundation of the NHS, attempted to rectify the unfortunate 'error' made by the Willink Committee by proposing an expansion in medical school output and the creation of new, provincial medical schools. It anticipated that the more serious part of medical education would occur after, not before, qualification, and that work in NHS hospitals would need to be combined with thorough postgraduate training. Undergraduate training would need to be broadened to include social studies and psychology, as well as the traditional subjects. The twelve London medical schools needed rationalisation, according to Todd, preferably by pairing them and integrating them into nearby colleges of London University. Finally, the report suggested that a new grade of hospital doctor was needed, to acommodate those who had passed through specialist training before a consultant job became available. This new post, of 'specialist', was effectively a consultant without a consultant's resources, in particular the all-important quota of hospital beds.

Only the proposal of a new grade caused real opposition, although all the others prompted criticism and resistance. Postgraduate education was an inevitability, given technological development and the pharmaceutical 'revolution'. Undergraduate education clearly needed updating, and the psychological sciences had to be given their due. Even the London medical schools could manage to combine, if not fuse with the University proper, since there was no insoluble conflict threatening the consultants' control over resources, or their interests in private medicine. The 'specialists' idea, on the other hand, challenged both power and privilege. What if the new 'specialists', effectively equal to consultants but without their power, sided with the NHS administration against the real consultants? What would happen if whole departments of 'specialists' were created? What if retiring consultants were replaced by new 'specialists', and control of beds reverted to the administration? What if all the new 'specialists' entered private medicine, too? The prospect was too frightening, and the consultants resisted firmly. Their compromise was an offer to increase the number of new consultant posts faster than the number of training posts, announced in the Godber Report in 1969. The spectre of 'specialists' vanished as the career bottleneck was eased.

The Salmon Reform

In contrast with the consultants, the nursing profession had to capture positions of power, not hold them. Since nursing had been shaped by the NHS in a way that medicine had not, and since nursing was women's work to medicine's manly craft, the prestige of nursing was low. So were nurses' incomes, and nursing was therefore a potential area for conflict within the health service. The options open to nurses seemed unsatisfactory. Either they could reject the submissiveness of the caring role and adopt a more confrontational attitude, or they could concentrate on their responsibilities to the ill and learn to tolerate the consequences. Trade unionism had a track record of improving incomes and working conditions, but largely in productive industries where industrial action hurt the employer rather than the consumer, and its implications for nursing were unacceptable to many nurses. The prospect of confrontation must also have alarmed young, mostly working class, women who had chosen nursing precisely because of its caring role, and who would come into conflict with powerful male administrators and doctors if they became militant. Professionalism, on the other hand, paid no bills, and that became increasingly important as both living standards and inflation rose in the sixties.

The Royal College of Nursing was able to resolve this dilemma in a way that the health workers' trade unions could not. The RCN's dominance in pay negotiation on the Whitley Council was matched by its base amongst Matrons and Senior Nursing staff, and its experience in nurse education and training. The trade unions had no comparable power base outside the mental hospitals, and no comparable experience in technical education for nursing. The RCN produced a blueprint for change in 1964 (*Administering the Hospital Nursing Service*) and this greatly influenced the Government committee that produced the Salmon Report (on Senior Nursing Staff structure) in 1966. This document was an attempt to boost nursing by introducing managerial methods, and dovetailed with the general desire at government level to incorporate workers into management decision-making in the health service. As the Salmon Report put it ...

> Nursing appears to occupy a secondary position. This stems from the incoherence of the nursing administration itself and a seeming inability on the part of nurses themselves to assert the rights of their emergent profession.

This managerialist perspective offered the nursing hierarchy a great deal. The Matrons had been largely excluded from the Hospital Management Committees. They had no authority over the new professions in health care that were open to women, like physiotherapy, radiography, and speech therapy. They had also lost control of catering, laundry and cleaning services to a new breed of departmental heads who were directly responsible to the lay Hospital Administrator. On their behalf, first the RCN and then the Salmon Report proposed an adminstrative structure for nursing that would match the administrative structure of hospital administration itself. The opportunity for senior nurses to influence resource allocation reappeared with the Salmon Report, and the timing could hardly have been better. Nurse-managers were proposed as part of the managerial solution to the problems of an expanding health service frequently forced to 'make do and mend', and they quickly acquired a new managerial language. The new ranks of senior nurses had to learn to distinguish between 'structural' and 'sapiential' authority; 'job description', 'job grading' and 'job specification'; and 'informative' and 'conclusive' conferences, amongst other professional mysteries.

At first sight the Salmon reform looks like the evolution of a pressure group within a state administration; in its responsiveness to the needs of Matrons and the top flight of the nursing hierarchy it was. In its adoption of a managerial style borrowed from commerce and private industry, it was a genuinely professional reform, enhancing the market value of nursing by concentrating on the management of labour and the labour process, rather than of patients and patient care. Perhaps it was that choice of labour management rather than patient care that made the Salmon Report's reception uneven, for pilot schemes to test the proposed structure were planned, to see if it would work. Nursing was 'saved' from this delay to its growth by the intervention of the same National Board for Prices and Incomes that had found the 'low earning opportunities' amongst ancillary workers.

Militant Professionalism

The NBPI had examined the issue of nurses' pay, in the light of the Salmon Report recommendations, for a year before it reported, in 1968. It awarded 14% increase to newly qualified nurses, and proportionately smaller increases to higher grades, dropping to 9% for the most senior nurses. More importantly, the NBPI recommended the nationwide introduction of the Salmon structure before the pilot schemes had been evaluated. The financial significance of the new structure matched the role of 'productivity' amongst NHS manual workers. A well-organised, and relatively well-paid, career ladder would act as a magnet to nurses needing to improve their living standards, and the pay differentials established could contribute to pay limitation in the future. The prospect of competitive advancement would reduce the pressure of pay demands *for all* from those who successfully climbed the ladder, and the ideology of professional service would allow the higher ranks to tolerate the low pay of their subordinates.

If that assessment had been correct, the RCN would have copied the medical professional, in which the consultants tolerated the long hours of work and relatively low pay of their junior staff very well throughout the sixties. In fact, nurses still needed to establish their professional power, and the RCN needed to retain its dominance over the rival trade unions. It had got its way over nurse-managers, and it now needed to show that it could win (or àt lest fight) over nurses' pay. When inflation threatened to undermine the 1968 awards, the RCN launched the 'Raise the Roof' campaign of 1969-70, appealing for public support for their pay campaign in the first demonstration of militant professionalism. Through the 'Raise the Roof' campaign, the RCN staked its place amongst the organisations fighting for a better deal for nurses, and showed that professionalism and weakness were no longer equivalents.

The third success for nursing professionalism in the sixties was that it survived the Salmon reform and continued to develop the art and craft of nursing proper, not just nurse-management. In theory the cadre of nurse-managers were subordinate to the practical workers, since their function was to provide appropriate resources and working conditions for nurses on the wards. In practice, prestige, power and income were divested away from the ward nurses, to their managers.

Patient care became less well-paid than nursing administration, and economic pressures drove enthusiastic and capable ward nurses away from patient contact, into purely managerial posts. The response within nursing and, with the RCN acting as facilitator, was to emphasise the caring role and systematise the nurse's work into the 'nursing process'.

The 'nursing process' theory concentrated on detailed analysis of the relationship between nurse and patient, with an emphasis on the nurse's accountability to the patient. A new language developed to describe this 'process', just as it had done in nurse management. The 'nursing process' became accepted wisdom in the seventies, and reinforced the trend towards professionalism in nursing as well as counterbalancing the bias towards management. If the doctor-patient relationship was the central idea in medical professionalism, then nursing could claim professional status by close attention to the 'nursing process'.

Hospital Scientific Service?

Medicine, as a profession, imposed its interests on the NHS. Nursing was changed by the state health service, but fought hard to fit itself to medicine's professional template. What would happen to the technical specialists who had either grown in numbers since 1948, or who had appeared only after the nationalisation of the hospitals? The medical laboratory technicians and the radiographers were the most numerous representatives of the former group; cardiology technicians, psychologists, nuclear medicine scientists, and biomedical engineers were among the newcomers. Each group had its own organisation, concerned with educational standards and the maintenance of registers of trained specialists, but none of them had professional bodies to match the BMA or the RCN. Technical workers in these specialist jobs often had low incomes, lacked promotional opportunities, and had little influence over policy decisions, even when these affected their work. Their place in health care was a frustrating one, despite their close connection with developments in medical science.

The moderniser's answer to the frustration of some 27,000 technicians in 30 or so different groups was given in the Zuckerman Report of 1968. A 'Hospital Scientific Service' was needed that included all these workers, giving them a career structure that would transcend specialist demarcations, and an administrative apparatus to coordinate scientific developments at local, regional and national level. New technical developments could be absorbed into the NHS, without the formation of a new professional group. Massed together, technical workers could aspire to greater influence in policy making than they had ever had when isolated in their small professional groups.

The Zuckerman Report envisaged a specialist career structure within a state organisation, perhaps equivalent to the hierarchic ladders of the Civil Service. Members of the Hospital Scientific Service would have no common educational origin, but would be grouped together to fit into the pattern of the developing health service. In that respect, the NHS staff could not constitute a professional group like medicine or nursing, where specialisation stemmed from a basic education, but they would correspond to a trade union concept of skilled workers organised within an industry.

For a number of reasons, the Hospitals Scientific Service never developed. It was a threat to the autonomy of existing, if feeble, professional organisations, and it hinted that industrial unionism might replace professional separatism. It posed problems of negotiating equivalence, relative rank, and parity, and these were to sour relations between groups of workers. Pay restraint prevented substantial, across-the-board increases that could have smoothed out the uneveness in pay and conditions, and re-organisation of the NHS in 1974 pre-empted the creation of a highly-centralised structure for scientific services. Of all the modernising reforms, the Zuckerman Report's proposals were probably both the best and the least realistic. The HSS would have organised scientists, and technicians, in a rational way, inside a State industry. As a project, it fitted into the Fabian idea of a wise and well-ordered administrative machine dispensing health care. It had no lasting place in the reality of the NHS, which remained the battleground between conflicting ideas and social orders that it had been at its birth in June 1948.

Medicalisation

Centralisation of health services, and increasingly efficient management, were presented in the sixties as the necessary preconditions for effective modern medical care. Medical care was certainly effective. People recovered from meningitis, when previously they would have died. Tuberculosis could be treated with medication rather than surgery, whilst the infected individual carried on living a normal life instead of disappearing to a sanitorium. Malignant diseases became treatable by surgery and drug therapy, and whilst the results overall were not too good, some were impressive. The quality of life, more than its duration, was being altered by the new science, and for many who used the NHS the change was for the better. But not for all.

If medical intervention was a solution to some problems, its value to others was questionable, and at times it seemed to be the cause, not the cure, of illness. The rapid incorporation of maternity care into the hospitals was nearly complete by 1970, and the provision of obstetric skills for all, or almost all, pregnant women was welcome to many and essential to some. Yet both the rate and pattern of obstetric intervention seemed to be determined by factors other than the medical needs of pregnant and labouring women. In 1970 the desire of hospital obstetricians to eliminate midwifery services run by local authorities was expressed in the Peel Report, which suggested that hospital midwives could undertake domiciliary confinements in certain circumstances, as well as undertake antenatal care in GP surgeries. The obstetricians did not want to wait until the local authority health services were absorbed into the NHS, in the 1974 reorganisation – they wanted immediate action! Was this enthusiasm simply a response to complicated pregnancies and disasters in labour? Or was it part of 'empire-building', a measure of the struggle for resources within the NHS? Was it a sign that rational planning to meet needs was overwhelmed by professionals' preoccupation with the scarcity of funds, staff and equipment?

Pregnancy and labour became mechanised as well as more medically-controlled. Induction of labour, monitoring of contractions and the baby's heart, ultra-sound scanning to measure foetal growth – all contributed to improving the safety of pregnancy, and the scientific content of obstetrics. Yet the new science was not tested, carefully taught, and slowly disseminated. On the contrary, it was rapidly applied, often by inexperienced or inadequately trained staff, in massive, unplanned experiments involving women who were unaware of their experimental role. In the seventies it was recognised that obstetric intervention had gone too far, too fast, and that it caused problems as well as solving them. By then some of the women who had been experimental subjects had reacted against their treatment, and created a movement that was to challenge 'modern' obstetrics. Was all the scientific enthusiasm just a simple response to the problems of pregnancy and child-birth? Were the machines and the new techniques the tangible outcome of a struggle for scarce resources, and the mechanised labour part of the politics of health? Did some of the enthusiasm for science come from the machine-makers themselves, who needed orders now so that they could work on the next generation of profitable monitors, pumps and scanners?

Abortion Law Reform

If commerce had a role in medical progress, so too did 'crime'. Redefinition of criminality and deviance was part of sixties modernisation, and reform of the Abortion laws joined changes in the laws on divorce, homosexuality, capital punishment and drug abuse. In itself, abortion law reform had been a target for socialist and feminists since the brief but powerful alliance between women and the labour movement immediately after the First World War. The Abortion Law Reform Campaign (ALRA) had been the main pressure group, and Private

Members' Bills in 1953, 1961, 1965 and 1966 had marked the reformers' unsuccessful offensives. Modification, rather than wholesale reform, of the law had occurred, and legal abortions were permitted in exceptional circumstances, when a pregnant woman's mental or physical health was seriously threatened. By 1967 just under 10,000 abortions were performed each year within the NHS, and the same number were carried out privately. No one knew how many illegal abortions were performed, but that did not prevent many guessing, and their estimates ranged between 15,000 and 100,000 a year. Illegal abortions could end with haemorrhage, infection, infertility and, occasionally, the death of the aborted woman. The availability of abortion depended on the interpretation of the law by gynaecologists, and such interpretation seemed sensitive to women's ability to meet private fees. Legal clarity was needed, and some way of reducing the numbers of illegal abortions seemed necessary, if only to reduce the numbers of casualties needing treatment.

The chance for reform came with another Private Member's Bill, introduced to the House of Commons by the Liberal MP David Steel, in 1966. This Bill enabled the Liberals to join Labour in the process of social modernisation, at a time when the Liberals were seeking a breakthrough that would restore some of their old power. (A decade later they were still trying, this time through the 'Lib-Lab' pact, but with the aim of retaining rather than initiating social advances). For Labour it was an addition to their range of reforms, and they could afford to be benevolently neutral. If it succeeded, Labour would stress that benevolence and welcome reform. If it was opposed, and failed, Labour's neutrality would allow them to escape the defeat. Feminists, hoping for more liberal laws that might make access to abortion easier and more equitable, could not afford to oppose Steel's Bill, although its real intention was far from feminist (and socialist) objectives. The right of women to control their fertility was not an issue in Steel's Bill, since abortion was seen as a medical solution to marginal social problems involving maladjusted, ill and inadequate individuals. These people – epileptics (!), women in prison, persistent offenders, women who had neglected their children, drug addicts, alcoholics, women with excessively large families, wives of drunkards and ne'er-do-wells – needed firm but compassionate help from a 'caring' society, rather than persecution as criminals. 'Severe social hardship' was to be the reason for aborting a pregnant woman, not her desire to end the pregnancy. Illegal abortion had to be eliminated, of course, but access to legal abortion had to be controlled by careful legal definition and unchallengeable medical authority. Medicine was to be used openly as a form of social control, to sort out those who could not fit into satisfactory places in a fundamentally good society. For the modernisers, abortion law reform was needed to improve the social order, whilst for the right it was part of a eugenicist policy, aimed at reducing the fertility of the feckless poor.

The passage of Steel's Bill, as the 1967 Abortion Act, had an effect comparable to the 1948 NHS Act. Demand for services was much greater than expected; legal abortions increased from 35,000 in 1967 to 95,000 in 1971. The liberalisation of the law had exposed the real need for abortion services, and this had two dangerous consequences for modernising reformers and conservatives alike. If large numbers of women wanted or needed abortions, the problem of unwanted pregnancy was not so marginal, and the assumption that modernisation of the mixed economy could produce an essentially good, just and stable society was threatened. If, on the other hand, the women having abortions were not 'problem-cases' at all, then abortion was being used as a form of birth control, and this choice of contraceptive method was being made by the women themselves. If they were not 'problems', why did they not use cheaper (but more profitable) forms of contraception like the Pill? The wider use of abortion suggested that the women themselves were beginning to control their use of contraceptive methods, rather than accept the medically-approved choice of method, and this challenged the conventional distribution of power. Worse still, women accustomed to controlling their own fertility might want to control other aspects of their lives, like work and child-care, and neither the mixed economy nor its social structure could withstand such a challenge to inequality.

The subsequent opposition to the 1967 Abortion Act grew out of this political panic, and Labour, Conservative and Liberal MPs attempted to make the Act more restrictive, to prevent the 'abuse' of abortion on demand. The religious right spearheaded public campaigning against the 1967 Act with moral slogans about the sanctity of life, the naturalness of female subordination, and the importance of punishing sinners. (One of the saws of gynaecology was that 'good girls get fibroids and bad girls get babies'; retribution stalks *all* women, in that outlook). Their role, however, was as catalyst and organiser of a response that united different perspectives, just as ALRA's pressure for abortion law reform had done during the previous thirty years.

Thalidomide and the Power of the Drug Companies

Commerce, medicine and crimes of a different kind combined in another way, in the sixties. The West German company Chemie Grunenthal had first marketed a sedative, for use as a sleeping tablet, called Contergan, in 1957. It was then launched on the international market and sold by licensees in more than forty countries outside the socialist bloc. The British distributor was the Distillers Company, and it marketed this new drug under the name Distaval, emphasising its safety compared with the barbiturate sleeping tablets then widely used. Distaval became better known for its dangers than its safety, and by its chemical name – Thalidomide. Thalidomide was a genuinely new drug, and it had not been fully tested for side-effects before being marketed. Drug-testing regulations in West Germany were minimal at the time, and the drug's marketed status was used to project it into other countries with much more stringent regulations, like the USA.

When serious side-effects appeared, the manufacturers failed to respond to them rapidly, and even seemed to avoid acknowledgement of the drug's dangers. Nerve damage in those who took Thalidomide was the first side-effect noted, but the drug's ability to damage human embryos was what made it infamous and accelerated its withdrawal from the market. The deformed, almost limbless, babies born to mothers who had taken the safe drug Thalidomide were the price of pharmaceutical 'progress', and the unacceptable face of capitalism in health care. Whilst the pharmaceutical industry worldwide learned to be more careful, after the Thalidomide tragedy, it has never been able to escape its dilemma entirely. The Opren scandal in the eighties demonstrated that making profits sometimes means cutting corners, and the recipients of treatment may become the victims of experimental accidents.

The optimism of the sixties did not last, and the 'revolution' in health care slowed down as money ran out, as doubts about the motives of professionals and the value of their skills grew, and as health politics became public issues. The answers, from within the state, were to try more of the same – tighter control, better management, more efficiency, and greater effectiveness. Priorities became the key concern of the seventies, and resistance to change by those with low priority became a new feature of health politics. In the end, 'more of the same' facilitated a shift to the right and allowed a radical change of policy, in health care and social policy generally. We do not yet know if the resistance to change of the seventies can become a commitment to change in the eighties.

CHAPTER 4

Inequalities and Priorities

Britain's economic problems got worse, not better, in the seventies. New challenges to Britain's market position came from the Commonwealth countries, adding to the pressure from Germany, Japan and the USA, and prompting an economic realignment with the Common Market. Mass unemployment returned, with half a million (2.5% of the workforce) out of work in 1970, and $1\frac{1}{4}$ million (5.4%) unemployed by 1979. Employment in manufacturing industries fell by 17% during the decade. Inflation rates in consumer prices were higher than in other countries, with annual rises of 11.8% in the 10 years from 1968 to 1978 compared with 7.6% in the OECD countries. Capital export continued, with increasing economic reliance on overseas earnings and further erosion of the national industrial base. Manufactured goods were imported at an increasing rate; between 1968 and 1978 their volume, as a proportion of home market sales, rose by an annual average of 5.8%. In 1979, imported manufactured goods took 15.7% of the home market. Investments in domestic production declined. One brief attempt at the expansion of home industry, through credit extension engineered by the 1970-74 Conservative government, fizzled out in a property boom and rising inflation.

Only in 1979 did government responses change. Until then both Conservative and Labour government still believed that they could combine industrial modernisation at home with British economic power overseas. Familiar formulae were applied, although without great success. Attempts were made to reduce government borrowing by limiting government spending on public services, so that capital could be freed for industrial investment. Efforts were made to boost profits by cutting labour costs, through reduction in the power of trades unions to defend incomes and industries. The 1970-74 Conservative government opted for legal controls on trade union activity, and a policy of confrontation with militant unions (like the miners), but was beaten. Its successors, the Labour administrations of Wilson and Callaghan, chose to manipulate trade union loyalties through voluntary wage restraints, yet could not survive a conflict with low-paid workers in the winter of 1978-79. Margaret Thatcher's victory in the May 1979 election marked a change in strategy. The twin-track policy of home investment *and* capital export was abandoned. De-industrialisation and rising unemployment are now to be accepted as inevitable. Economic re-expansion, on a much more limited basis, has been postponed until uncompetitive industry has been annihilated or reformed from within. Trade union resistance to job-loss and industrial decline is to be smashed by unemployment backed by a reserve of legal powers. Capital export continues, and the economic balance within Britain is to shift from the industrial to the service and commercial sectors.

The NHS had its own twin-track policy throughout the seventies, and continues to do so in the early eighties, despite the change in government strategy. The themes of efficiency and effectiveness had become increasingly important at the beginning of the decade. Both Labour and Conservative governments sought to extend the NHS *and* strictly control its cost to the Exchequer. Labour, particularly under Health Ministers like Richard Crossman, emphasised the importance of directing resources to areas of greatest need. The Conservatives emphasised economic restraints within the NHS and encouraged pursuit of non-government finance for health, mainly through increasing private medicine.

'Efficiency' in administration reached its high point in the 1974 reorganisation of the NHS administration. Local authority health clinics were taken over by the health service, which itself was brought under the control of a three-tier administrative structure. The Department of Health sat at the summit of the new apparatus, and produced overall policy for the service. The three subordinate levels, of Region, Area and District, applied the policies handed down to them. By a process of 'delegation downward' and 'accountability upwards' a command structure was created in which Districts were subordinate to Areas, and Areas to Regions. Membership of the Regional, Area and District management bodies was determined by selection, although local government and trades union representation was automatic. The balance of power on the new Health Authorities was shared between (mostly medical) professionals and lay members from commercial backgrounds. Health Service Management, apart from the Authorities themselves, was dominated by uneasy coalition of full-time administrators often recruited straight from business schools, and senior professionals from medicine and nursing. This hierarchic structure matched that of business management and reflected comparable hierarchies in medicine and nursing. It was to become the basic instrument for enforcing DHSS, and therefore government, policy. The limited role for popular representation, through local government and union representation on Health Authorities, emphasised that 'need' was to be defined by professionals and administrators, and that government requirements were to over-ride other considerations. Even the new public watch-dog committees, the Community Health Councils, were charged with the task of conveying District Health Authority decisions to the local population, and were therefore one component of the command structure.

Labour's hope was that this efficient command structure would allow central government to impose standards on the NHS, and redirect resources within it, despite local opposition from health professionals or the public. The sixties preoccupation with management efficiency had provoked debate about clinical effectiveness. The Health Service may be well run, but did it work? Were people getting good treatment, when they needed it? Investigating clinical effectiveness led to the official rediscovery of inequalities in health and health care provisions. Class inequalities had been the staple diet of the left generally since the Industrial Revolution, but only became important to the state when Labour did, or potentially could, form governments. Labour's challenge to Conservatism, in the sixties and seventies, based on its promise to modernise the economy, also allowed it to talk of modernising the society by modifying class inequalities.

Health and Class

Class differences in health and illness, exposed by investigative sociology in the late sixties and the early seventies, came under government scrutiny through a working party chaired by the

President of the Royal College of Physicians, Sir Douglas Black. The *Black Report*, published (and nearly smothered at birth) by the Conservative government in 1980, detailed the impact of illness in a class society..

Whilst everyone's health and expectation of life have improved since the beginnings of state-run health care, the difference between classes have been preserved and in some cases, widened. The frequency rates of premature death in men from different social classes are shown in Figure 6. The unskilled workers fare worse than average, and much worse than professional workers of the same age. The gap between the wealthiest and the poorest has widened, with the unskilled worker much more likely than the professional worker to die before retirement from lung cancer, strokes, heart disease, road traffic accidents, stomach and duodenal ulcers, and stomach cancer. If we take the health expectations of professional workers as the normal expectation, the health of unskilled

Figure 6
Mortality of Men by Occupational Class, 1930-1972

SMR (Standardised Mortality Ratios)

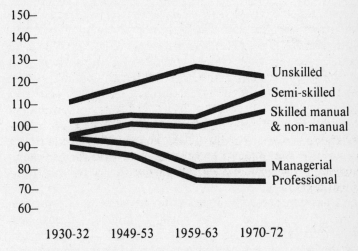

Source: P. Townsend and N. Davidson, *Inequalities in Health*, 1982.

Figure 7
Death Rates of Unskilled and Semi-skilled Male Workers Compared With Professional and Managerial Male Workers

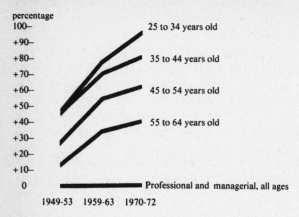

Source: P. Townsend and N. Davidson, *Inequalities in Health*, 1982.

Figure 8
Death Rates of Skilled Manual and Non-manual Male Workers Compared With Professional and Managerial Male Workers

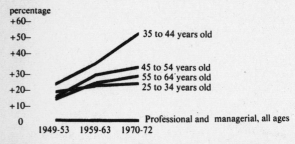

Source: P. Townsend and N. Davidson, *Inequalities in Health*, 1982.

workers has deteriorated relative to the professionals, as Figure 7 shows. This class gap in illness is not simply related to poverty, for skilled manual and non-manual workers on higher incomes than the unskilled show a similar, but smaller, gap as demonstrated in Figure 8.

The class gap exists throughout life. At birth and during the first month of life the risk of death in families of unskilled workers is double that of professional families, whilst babies born into the families of skilled manual workers run a risk one and a half times as great. In the first year of life the class gap widens. For every death of a male child in a professional family, two will die in skilled workers' families and three in the families of unskilled workers. The higher death rate in the working class families will be caused by more chest diseases and more accidents – both hazards that are directly related to the quality and safety of housing, the education of the parents, and the family income. Between 1 and 14 years, the class gap narrows, but is never abolished. Among boys the death rate in unskilled workers' families are twice as high as in professional families, and girls are one and a half times as high. After 15 years of age the class gap widens in early adult life, and narrow towards retirement. The next three figures show the class gap for heart and artery disease, diseases of the digestive system, and lung diseases.

Amongst women the class gap is narrower, but amongst women over 35 it has also widened since 1949. Women in unskilled or semi-skilled manual jobs, or married to men in such

Figure 9
The Class Gap in Heart and Arterial Disease

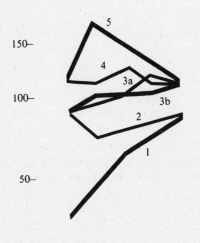

Mortality ratios,
(percentage)

5=unskilled

4=semi-skilled
3a=skilled non-manual
3b=skilled manual

2=managerial
1=professional

Source: P. Townsend and N. Davidson, *Inequalities in Health*, 1982.

Figure 10
The Class Gap in Diseases of the Digestive System

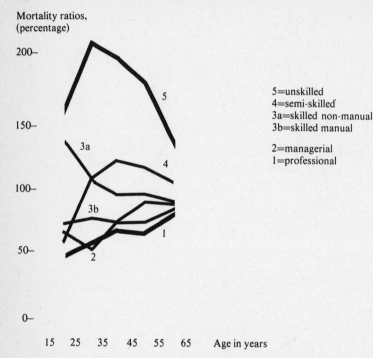

Mortality ratios,
(percentage)

5=unskilled
4=semi-skilled
3a=skilled non-manual
3b=skilled manual

2=managerial
1=professional

15   25   35   45   55   65   Age in years

Source: P. Townsend and N. Davidson, *Inequalities in Health*, 1982.

jobs, have a higher death rate from diseases of the heart and arteries, lung diseases, and infections, than professional women. The risk of death in child-birth declined by a third during the sixties, but women in the unskilled working class were twice as likely to die as were professional women. The class gap reverses only with deaths from malignant diseases and mental illness, when women in professional and managerial jobs have the higher risk.

Use of the NHS also varies between the classes and the services available to different social classes are themselves different in quality and quantity. For example, unskilled and semi-skilled workers visit their general practitioner more often than their professional equivalents, but less often than they need

Figure 11
The Class Gap in Lung and Other Respiratory Diseases

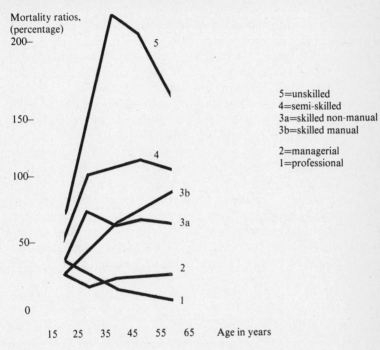

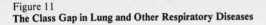

Source: P. Townsend and N. Davidson, *Inequalities in Health*, 1982.

to, given their experience of illness and health hazards. Women from the lowest income groups make less use of antenatal and family planning services yet run the highest risks of infant illness and death, maternal death in childbirth, and unintended pregnancy. The class gap also exists for cancer of the cervix, which is much more likely to kill working class women than the professional women who are most likely to have screening tests for cervical cancer.

Other preventive services, like dentistry, are used less by the working class than by professionals, and the quality of service available to working people tends to be lower. For the elderly, publicly-provided services fail to compensate for differences in income, let alone differences in need. A study published in 1965 showed that half the retired people from managerial and professional backgrounds had privately-paid or local authority domestic help, and nearly half the remainder said they needed such help. Only one in six of those from unskilled manual working class backgrounds who were severely incapacitated had any domestic help from outside the family, and only one in five of the remainder felt they needed help.

The hospital services to which the trade unions sought access in the forties are used more by the working class. Skilled, semi-skilled and unskilled workers and their families occupy proportionately more hospital beds, and make greater use of outpatient and casualty departments, than do employers, managers, and professional workers. This usage reflects the greater risks of accident and injury at work and at home, and the higher rates of serious illness experienced by the working population, and possibly their low uptake of preventive services. Yet despite the greater use and need for hospital services by the working class population, their availability is determined by the distribution of professional and managerial workers. A study of the fifteen NHS Regions in the early seventies showed that the amount spent on hospitals and community health services was closely related to the proportion of professional and managerial workers in the Region's population. The more affluent the Region was, the more money it spent on health service. The more semi-skilled and unskilled workers it served, the lower its spending!

A survey conducted later in the decade in three areas of council housing produced a similar picture. The areas were an East London Borough with a long history of deprivation, a middle class estate in the Midlands, and a 'problem' estate, also in the Midlands. There was much in common between the working class areas, but the important finding, in terms of provision of health services, was that 'a working class person is at a greater disadvantage if he [sic] lives in a predominantly working class area than if he lived in a socially mixed area'. (Skrimshire, *Area Disadvantage, Social class and the Health Service*, Oxford, 1978)

The Inverse Care Law

Julian Tudor Hart summed up the maldistribution of health services in the 'Inverse Care Law', which is rarely quoted in full because of its political conclusions. Here it is:

> In areas with most sickness and death, general practitioners have more work, larger lists, less hospital support, and inherit more clinically ineffective traditions of consultation, than in the healthiest areas; and hospital doctors shoulder heavier case-loads with less staff and equipment, more obsolete buildings, and suffer recurrent crises in the availability of beds and replacement staff. These trends can be summed up as the Inverse Care Law: that the availability of good medical care tends to vary inversely with the need of the population served.
>
> If the NHS had continued to adhere to its original principles, with construction of health centres a first priority in industrial areas, all financed from taxation rather than direct flat-rate contribution, free at the time of use, and fully inclusive of all personal health services, including family planning, the operation of the Inverse Care Law would have been modified much more than it has been; but even the service as it is has been effective in redistributing care, considering the powerful social operating against this. If our health services had evolved as a free market, or even on a fee-for-item-of-service basis prepaid by private insurance, the law would have operated much more completely than it does; our situation might approximate that in the United States, with the added disadvantage of smaller national wealth. The force that creates and maintains the Inverse Care Law is the operation of the market, and its cultural and ideological superstructure which has permeated the thought and directed the ambitions of our profession during all of its modern history. The more health services are removed from the force of the market, the more successful we can be in redistributing care away from its "natural" distribution in a market economy; but this will be a redistribution, an intervention to correct a fault natural to our form of society, and therefore incompletely successful and politically unstable, in the absence of more fundamental social change. (*The Lancet*, 27.2.71)

The role of market forces is crucial. If spending on health services favours the affluent, it does so because of the special realtionship between the affluent and the controllers of health care, the professionals.

Firstly, the affluent and the professional traditionally share power in the NHS. In the mid-1960s a review of Regional Hospital Board membership showed that 64% were doctors (mostly consultants), and only one industrial worker was found amongst 108 members of boards studied in detail. Eleven of the chairmen of the fifteen Regional Boards were either directors, partners or chairmen in one or more of fifty different companies. Members of Regional Boards not only made policy, but often enacted it on Hospital Management Committees as well. The review found that 21% of HMC Chairmen came from RHBs with:

> 4 Lord Lieutenants, 20 deputy Lieutenants, 146 JPs, 12 peers or baronets, 5 wives, widows or offspring of peers, 1 retired ambassador, 1 ex-Lord Mayor, 8 retired admirals or generals. Of a sample of 92 of the HNCs, one quarter of the chairmen were company directors and not a single one as far as was known was a wage-earner. (John Robson, 'NHS Incorporated', *International Journal of Health Services*, Vol. 3 No. 3 1973).

The 1974 administrative reform did little to alter the dominance of this social élite and its alied commercial interests in the control of the service, although it may have incorporated a larger trade union and local government component into decision-making.

Secondly, the affluent and the medical profession (and probably the top layers of nursing and other health professions) have a common social origin. Recruitment to medical schools concentrated on the output of public and grammar schools in the sixties, and still favours students from professional backgrounds, despite the growth of comprehensive education. Medicine remains a self-selecting profession, at many levels. The children of doctors are disproportionately represented in that medical school entrance, and have the advantage of already being partly socialised into professional values and attitudes. Education for conformity is promoted through training programmes based on emulation of 'excellence' and through hierarchic and highly competitive career-structures.

Finally, affluence and medicine share the cash nexus of 'liberal professionalism'. Private practice, at least for hospital consultants, *may* be important financially, but is *always* important ideologically. It brings together individuals usually of similar culture, in a fixed and unambiguous relationship of provider and customer, within a context of time, courtesy and respect. The contrast with socialised medicine could not be greater. Medical work within the NHS can be rushed and cramped, conducted with disagreeable people who cannot reward doctors personally for the discomfort they inflict upon them, in circumstances that demand greater skills than those the doctors possess. No wonder that private medicine holds such attraction, and is defended as a matter of principle within the profession. It is a refuge from the conflicts that arise in highly stratified societies, where artificial inequalities (of ability) are promoted as natural, and real inequalities (of need) are denied. The extent to which this 'liberal professionalism' survives, even after three decades of state health care, should teach us one lesson. The extent to which an alternative philosophy, based on ideas of 'service', sympathy and even soldarity, coexists within professionalism, teaches us another. This coexistence appears within the structure of the health service, shaping the distribution of public resources to fit the landscape of private interest. Figure 12 compares resource distribution with the distribution of merit awards of consultants. Merit awards are bonuses paid to consultants, by fellow-consultants, in secret. They tend to go disproportionately to part-time consultants in specialities with ample private practice, and are densely distributed in the private sector's richest territory – London and

Figure 12
Resources and Merit Awards, by Region

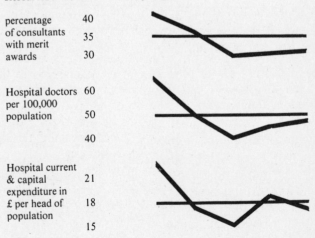

Source: John Robson, *Quality, Inequality and Health Care*, 1977

the Home Counties. Health service resources tend to follow the powerful professionals, who in turn follow the cash nexus. Whilst the NHS succeeded in redistributing *some* public resources towards areas of greatest need, it has modified the picture but not painted a new one.

The coexistence of the cash nexus and the social provision of services ends at the limits of power. In the seventies every significant group of health workers took part in some kind of industrial action or agitation about income or work conditions, or both. Ancilliary staff, ambulance crews, radiographers and physiotherapists and nurses took to the streets, and began to withdraw labour, in disputes that reflected low pay, poor management and the accumulated years of under-funding. The organisations of professional workers, like the Royal College of Nursing, were careful to keep their grievances separate from the complaints of non-professionals and their unions. Professionals then were concerned to serve, saw the pay issue in an almost sordid light, and rejected industrial action in favour of appeals for fair play. The non-professionals, usually poorly paid, in low-status work and often recruited abroad for import as British 'Guest Workers' had not experienced fair play and did not expect much from it. Neither approach made very much headway. The greatest obstacle to improved pay rates was the continuation of incomes policies in one form or another, by both Conservative and Labour governments. Even the doctors were to suffer pay restraint, and their response was to rediscover trades union militancy.

The Decade of Discontent

The first round of industrial disputes lasted from 1972 to 1976. The Conservatives' Counter-Inflation Act (1972) required a pay pause, and in practice this broke the traditional connection between pay rates for NHS ancilliary workers and local government manual workers. The trade unions representing NHS ancilliary staff responded by launching a selective strike wave that involved 750 hospitals at its height. The union campaign failed to break pay restraint, but it reinforced the changes in local union organisation, and in local union-management relations, that had begun in the sixties, and made further industrial action both more likely. Pay restraint interrupted the negotiation of nursing pay in 1972, and limited increases in 1973-4 to below levels acceptable to either the RCN or unions like COHSE and NUPE. The first national campaign of industrial action by nurses began in April 1974, with the RCN retaining the dominant role that it had won through the 1969 'Raise the Roof' agitation. By 1974 the RCN had evolved a steward system, and began to use it to mobilise for mass resignation (a professional's way of walking off the job, copied from the BMA) and for mass demonstrations. The main union rival to the RCN was COHSE, which had suffered the disgrace of expulsion from TUC in 1971 for its failure to oppose the Conservatives' Industrial Relations Act. Its base amongst nurses was mainly in the large mental illness and mental handicap hospitals, and it was able to restore some of its trade union credibility through the direct action its nursing members took in those hospitals.

The nurses' pay campaign, along with the third stage of the Heath government's incomes policy, was inherited by a Labour administration. The new Labour government continued its predecessor's pay policy, and used a special commission of inquiry to resolve the specific problem. The inquiry's findings noted the familiar story of health workers' incomes: pay had fallen behind comparative occupations; a significant pay increase was needed; and the differential scale needed simplifying if it was to survive. The pay increase was agreed, and named the Halsbury award, after the commission's chairman. 'Halsbury' was to become the benchmark for the next conflict over nurses' pay, in 1982, and another upswing in the repetitive rise and fall of health service pay rates.

The aggressiveness and trade union style learned by the RCN was picked up by the medical profession. The BMA did not initiate the militant professionalism of the hospitals doctors' strike of 1975-6, for it was preoccupied with a much more important issue – Labour's threat to private medicine. Public debate about private practice and its impact on the NHS had been turned into a major conflict, both through local union action and Labour Party design. The campaign against private medicine had a number of consequences, (described in Chapter Five), but it certainly acted as an alternative issue to pay problems within NHS unions, and allowed a defensive Labour Party to launch an attack on the Conservatives and the medical profession. It also kept the BMA busy, and when a new contract was negotiated for junior hospital doctors, the BMA misread the mood of the doctors completely.

Unofficial industrial action of various kinds developed amongst hospital doctors, and spread across the country, involving 11,000 medical staff at the height of the campaign. This dispute developed despite the BMA, not because of it, and it challenged Labour's pay policy. The planned new contract proposed basic pay scales for a 40 hour working week, and overtime rates for extra hours. Because of pay restraint, there was little extra money available to fund overtime payments, and these worked out at ludicrously low levels, since the *average* working time of junior doctors was 80 hours a week! The BMA had always got its priorities right, and had tolerated this situation extremely well. The unofficial dispute, and its challenge to Labour, made the BMA realise that its flagging campaign in defence of private medicine could be reinforced, if it could recruit the junior doctors' support. The pay issue suddenly became important, and part of a two-pronged attack on the Labour government. The Labour administration wisely settled the pay issue by allowing some local flexibility in negotiating the contentious overtime rates, and separated the two prongs of the BMA attack. At local level consultants and juniors jointly negotiated the most favourable overtime payments possible, and broke the pay policy without being seen to do so.

The whole episode threatened to undermine the acceptability of the Review Body system for determining doctors' pay. The Review Body had acquiesced over Labour's pay restraint when applied to the junior doctors' new contract, had done the same to the 1974 pay award, and in 1973 had accepted Conservative incomes policy as its limits too. Prior to these demonstrations of its subordinacy, the whole 1969 Review Body had resigned when the Labour government had referred the Review body award to the National Board for Prices and Incomes. The Heath government recruited a new Review Body, in 1971, but the message had been understood, and for the next few years the 'independent' Review Body became part of the pay restraint machinery.

It was during this period that the medical profession came closest to an internal crisis. The junior hospital doctors not only undertook industrial action, including withdrawal of labour, but also rejected the Review Body in principle, and refused to give evidence on pay to it for three years after their dispute. The question of TUC affiliation surfaced inside the BMA (although not for long), just as it kept doing inside the RCN, as members drew their own conclusions from the new-found militancy. In the end both the BMA and the RCN were able to survive this attack on their autonomy from the labour movement. For the BMA, survival was easy, given the profession's natural alliance with Conservatism, and the renewal of ancillary worker militancy in 1979. Inside the RCN the situation was different, and the challenge to insular professionalism stronger. It was not until the end of another long pay campaign, in 1982, that the RCN became safe from trade unionism proper.

In 1979 yet another NHS pay dispute ended, and soon afterwards the Callaghan administration was replaced by a Conservative government that began to change the rules. A shift to the right occurred within the country, particularly within the working class in the affluent South East. The low pay campaign of 1978-79 certainly pitched the TUC against the Labour government, but this further bout of industrial action was the detonator, not the charge, that brought down Labour. The 'old' methods, sponsored by Labour in the sixties, and carried on by Tory and Labour alike in the seventies, did not seem to work, and something really new was needed. This also became true of the politics of health, in 1979.

The winter pay offensive against Labour's 5% pay limit had enrolled NHS ancillary staff, and the ambulance service. The ancillary workers' unions claimed that inflation combined with pay rises for comparable workers in other industries had effectively returned ancillary pay levels to their 1970 level. The ambulance crews presented a special case in that their pay levels should have been related to other emergency services, but had declined relatively. The dispute inside the NHS ended with the inevitable commission, which this time examined pay comparability. the commission partially supported the ambulance crews' claim, but not the ancillary workers, who reacted very positively to the 12% demand in 1982 because of this dismissal. Whilst looking at nurses' pay, the Comparability Commission found that the lower job grades deserved the highest increases, whilst the higher echelons of nurse-management deserved smaller increments, or even no increase at all in some cases. The same applied to other professional groups, confirming the principle that the hierarchic career structures of the sixties had contributed to the persistence of low pay rates. The Commission also noted that there was 'no coherent approach to pay' inside the NHS, with doctors referring to a Review Body, nurses negotiating through a Whitley Council whose management representatives had different policies from their equivalents on other NHS Whitley Councils, whilst administrators compared themselves to Civil Service grades. Coherence had never been a strong feature of the health service, outside the political rhetoric of uncritical Labour supporters and of backwoodsmen on the right. Many planners, politicians and professionals had pursued coherence as a goal, but just as the issue of a rational pay structure for the NHS became officially debatable, with all the implications that held for professionalism and unionism, Thatcher's administration took office.

The Planners' Decade

The national planning of health workers' pay scales never took off, but other kinds of inequalities were attacked by the planners of the newly-reorganised NHS. Inequalities in the provision of services, and in the patterns of health and illness of different classes, became legitimate targets for planners keen to deploy resources in the most effective way. Serious, large-scale health care planning began in the seventies, with the aim of reducing the disparities between the most and least needy in Britain, and the credibility of modernisation, within a mixed economy, hinged on this socially just perspective. The drive for rational planning also recognised, in a roundabout way, the political rivalries and traditions that had guided the growth of the NHS, and attempted to supercede them, by consensus. The mixed economy would work, the society built upon it could be made equitable and socially just (if not socialist), and sectional interests, like class antagonisms, could be absorbed into a style of work that smothered conflict and promoted harmonious compromise. This strategy has been weakened because its foundation, the mixed economy, has failed to work as hoped, and its practical manifestations inside the NHS have become sources of damage rather than renewal, and conflict rather than harmony. Nevertheless, both the overall strategy and its tactical expressions in health care were positive innovations that challenged the 'plague of custom' that had infected the NHS from its first day. The principle methods of the planners were incorporated into planning-cycles and priority planning; reallocation of resources according to measured need; and, finally (and most damaging) cash limits.

The NHS planning cycle, launched as a necessary adjunct to the structural reform of 1974, was designed to modify the pattern of health care, not by altering clinical judgements, but by imposing priorities for spending on clinical services. The DHSS collated the policies evolved in the fifties and sixties into *Priorities for Health and Personal Social Services in England*, a document published in 1976. This stated the government's priorities for development in the NHS, and was introduced as the touchstone of the new planning cycle. Regional and Area Health Authorities were to produce Strategic Plans, covering 10-15 year spans, and Area and District Health Authorities were to use these to produce annually-updated, three year projections for local developments. Central to both Strategic and Local Plans was a programme budget, which allocated money according to the published priorities of the DHSS.

In practice, the planning cycle was as ambitious and unrealistic as the hospital building programmes of the sixties. Relatively few plans have been produced, and arguably there has been more paper produced than progress. A lack of planning skills within the NHS administration, the need to sort out the confusion left by the 1974 structural reform and, in some Health Authorities, the need to cope with a limited budget and ever-costlier services, reduced the responsiveness of NHS managers to DHSS priorities and planning demands. The planning cycle was also complex, overambitious and difficult to operate, and was understandbly treated as unrealistic. It was also unacceptable to those given low priority, and their countervailing pressure was sometimes enough to divert resources away from services nominated as 'high priority'. With these limitations, the planning approach had to be modified, if it was to survive. The main change, which was encouraged by the Conservatives after 1979, was a shift from quantitative planning at DHSS level to the 'interpretation' of national guidelines by local Health Authorities. The idea that, say, the number of mental illness hospital day places should increase by x% over a given period was replaced by encouragement to develop day care for the mentally ill, allowing the existing power relationships to resolve problems of quantity and quality rather than submit to central edict. Given the dominance of professional interests in decision-making, particularly at ground level, and the particular power of professionals in those sectors of the NHS that are already best-funded, local 'interpretation' favours the status quo, rather than planned new development.

Changing Priorities

The political complexities of planning in the seventies become even more obvious when priority areas are examined in detail. 'Primary care', including general practitioner services, was identified as essential to any approach to preventing illness, yet proved virtually unplannable. The independent contractor status of doctors, dentists, pharmacists and opticians disallowed the budgetary manipulation that formed the basis of NHS planning. All that was left were exhortations, appeals to professional honour (in the mistaken belief that this was relevant to health care) and modifications to 'carrot and stick' inducements of the kind introduced by the 1966 Charter. Both the Report of the Royal Commission on the NHS (1979) and the Acheson Report on Primary Care in Inner London (1981) were to juggle these responses in their recommendations, but neither offered any forceful mechanism for change. In the absence of a real preventive strategy, the DHSS could only say 'look after yourself' to the population, in its booklet, *Prevention and Health: Everybody's Business*. The professionals who were literally in the business of health care were not seen as being responsible and acountable for preventive work, but people in general were, and the DHSS thereby exhausted its contribution to progress in primary care.

Attempts to plan developments in hospital services have been a drawn-out battle, given that the initial DHSS objective was to slow down the growth in current spending on surgery, medicine and maternity facilities, in order to fund higher priority areas. As we shall see, the planners had a weapon against unplanned expenditure, in the shape of cash-limited budgets, but in the end this had not proved to be strong enough. The acute and maternity services have been the main source of countervailing pressure on the planning cycle, and have effectively resisted demotion in the priority-table. By 1978 the DHSS had abandoned its earlier policy of cutting maternity facilities in favour of maintaining real levels of expenditure. The acute services intercepted resources intended for elsewhere; for example, the proportion of current and capital spending on mental illness services *fell* from 7.6% to 7.5% between 1975 and 1979, despite the high priority given to facilities for the mentally ill.

Maternity services, in planning terms, are the opposite side of the coin to general practice. Planners have come to primary care too soon, before even rudimentary centralisation has ocurred, and have been left with nothing much useful to do. In obstetrics, they have come too late, with little left to do except further reduce the rates of death and preventable handicap amongst newborn babies. Maternity care has become the most advanced area of modern medicine, in the sense that it adopted objectives and then achieved them. About 98% of babies are born in hospitals, with all the help (and, perhaps, hindrance) that 'science' can offer them. Because it is so advanced technically, obstetrics has become a political isue, in a more direct and aggressive way than it has been at any time since 1948. Perhaps this makes it the shape of things to come, for medicine as a whole? Its forwardness has also broken the professional consensus so often sought within the NHS. The Short Report on Perinatal Mortality (1980) advocated more obstetric technology. The Black report (1980) saw the solution to avoidable death and handicap in improving social conditions. The Conservatives saw that each advocated extra resources, and rejected both!

Society's Creditors

Health services, and general support, for the retired have always been advocated as necessary, but provision lagged behind promise as competition for limited funds intensified. Hospital services for the elderly in the seventies were targeted for extra capital spending, but their expansion was limited by counter demand from the acute services, and the general restriction of NHS budgets. Even the planned expansion in hospital facilities was seen as a minor component of necessary provision, in policy statements like the consultative document *A Happier Old Age*

(1978) and the Whtie Paper *Growing Older* (1981). Community-based care was to be the first line of provision for the increasing numbers of retired and elderly people, with the greater burden falling on local government.

Passing responsibility from the NHS to local authorities has a precedent almost as strong as the contrary movement of local authority health services into the centralised sector, in 1948 and 1974. The strategy of 'community care' is applied to large groups of people requiring extensive but low technology services, and permits the NHS to avoid budgeting for services that are expensive because they require a large workforce. This financial burden is shifted to local authorities, where no attempt to standardise services like home helps, meals-on-wheels, or day-centre care can be made, and where local political pressures can allow 'interpretations' of need to justify variations in provision. If the elderly were susceptible to the kind of technological intervention that exists in obstetrics, would not geriatrics have followed the same pattern as maternity services, with centralisation of provision under close medical supervision? The elderly offer no breakthrough in the kinds of medical care most favoured, even though medical and social services have much to offer older people with deteriorating health. They are therefore both unproductive and unprofitable, and so doubly unlikely to attract a proportionate share of funds and facilities. As local authorities themselves face budgetary restriction, their provision for the elderly infirm moves away from being a requirement, towards being one of several options. As the White Pater *Growing Older* put it: '... care in the community must increasingly mean care by the community ...'

Local authorities have also been left to deal with an increasing share of the problem of the mentally ill and mentally handicapped. Hospitals for both types of patients had been understaffed and underfunded since 1948, and a series of public scandals about maltreatment of patients and poor standards of care encouraged official idealisation of 'community care' for the mentally ill and handicapped as well. Provision of community facilities has rarely exceeded the reduction in hospital services. Training centre places for the adult mentally handicapped increased by 70% during the seventies, from just over 23,000 in 1969 to just under 39,000 in 1977, but expansion needed to increase to 223% of the 1969 level to reach the 1991 target of

75,000 places. Community residential facilities for mentally handicapped children were also outstripped by closure of hospital places for these children, with an increase of only 400 in the number of local authority residential places between 1969 and 1977.

The mentally ill were similarly treated. The 1962 Hospital Plan aimed to reduce the number of places in the massive asylum hospitals by half, by 1975. The target was reached by 1978, but the alternative facilities planned for District General Hospitals and endorsed in the 1975 White Paper *Better Services for the Mentally Ill* suffered from the general squeeze on hospital spending, and the decline in the hospital building programme. Local government provided day-centres, hostels and group homes for those with mental illnesses, according to local political and economic circumstances, but the emptying of the asylums contines almost regardless of circumstances, and by 1983 whole mental illness hospitals were threatened with closure. The response within the NHS to shrinking resources was, as ever, better management, expounded for mental illness services by the Nodder Report of 1980. Despite the piety of official proclamation and the honest endeavours of good Health Authorities, mentally ill people are drifting into the homeless, workless population that sleeps in cardboard boxes and derelict buildings, rumages through litter bins and provides police, courts and prisons with an unpunishable stratum of hopeless recidivists.

The second objective in planning health care in the seventies was to even-out spending across the country, and relate it to people's needs rather than custom or demand from within the health service. Finding a way to do this was the job of the Resource Allocation Working Party (RAWP), which was supposed to take into account measures of health needs, and social and environmental factors which affected the need for health care. The Working Party's final conclusions, in the RAWP Report, were published in 1976, demonstrating once again the obstacles to rational planning within a health service guided by considerations of power, not need.

The RAWP Report found that some Regional Health Authorities had up to 10% more money allocated to them than they deserved according to a complex formula of need, whilst others had up to 10% less. The formula was based on death rates within Regions, with allowance for the use made of health services by particular groups, like the elderly, women and young children. The Report argued that these disparities should be reduced gradually, by reallocating 'growth money' to the least-funded Regions, and this began in 1977-78. This meant that the overall growth rate in NHS spending of no more than 2% per year was modified according to Regional need, with 'poor' Regions (like Trent RHA) getting 4% compared with the 0.5% extra allocated to the 'rich' Thames Regional Health Authorities.

RAWP reveals the weakness of the managerial approach, and of the centralised control structure of the NHS. The Working Party had no measures of need available to it, other than the professional clinical judgements that had contributed to the disparities in funding. It therefore used the only data readily to hand – death rates – and assumed that these figures corresponded to the levels of illness and need for medical care within the Regions. The assumption is logical, and probably correct, but the point is that, nearly 30 years after its formation, the NHS had evolved no way of measuring needs other than by the crudest yardstick of life or death. That inability looks like a monstrous oversight to the architects of the service, and to the modernisers of sixties and seventies, yet it simply demonstrates that health professionals had been left to 'get on with the job' without too much outside scrutiny of the job itself. Market research might be fundamental to some industries, but health care had been organised according to political rather than productive criteria, and the outcome of health care was considered less important than the processes of curing and caring as described by the curers and carers.

In attempting to correct disparities, the RAWP Report made a second significant assumption. The money could be redistributed, but no allowance was made for its final use in providing specific services. Whether extra cash went to mental illness hospitals or geriatric day centres was to be decided through the planning cycle, even though that planning cycle was being rapidly undermined by resistance to change within the health service. Redistribution, in itself, was only intended to balance the Regions, and that will be its major achievement if it is continued through the eighties, despite the original intention of relating spending to needs.

Not only did the RAWP formula fail to relate spending to needs, but it was unable to incorporate measures of social deprivation like housing standards, income levels and unemployment, despite the accumulated evidence that they helped to make or break people's health. The justifcation used by the Working Party was that it was only concerned with correcting problems within the NHS, not within housing departments, social services, nor the local economy. Such insularity has its historic roots in the separation of the health service from local government, but does not prevent social circumstances from creating illness, nor discourage the NHS from shedding problems to local authorities!

The RAWP Report has become infamous for two reasons. It has reduced growth in funding in the four Thames Regions, where a dozen Teaching Hospitals and assorted specialist hospitals have been accustomed to high levels of finance. And it has penalised the most deprived areas within the allegedly rich Regions, for reduced funding has intensified competition for resources within these Regions, and displayed the balance of power within the NHS. With constricted budgets, difficult choices have had to be made in the kind of service provided. Should equipment and staff be centralised to a Teaching Hospital site, and District General Hospitals with community responsibilities shrunk, or even closed, to fund the shift? If the choice is extension of kidney dialysis facilities, or the closure of a crumbling Poor Law Infirmary that provides in-patient care for elderly ill people but also needs massive and expensive repair, which should be chosen? The conflict over choices like these is the same as the struggle around priorities in the planning cycle, but more intense because the issue is selective closure rather than selective growth. For all its innovative features and progressive principles, the RAWP formula applied to a static or shrinking budget degenerated into robbing Peter to pay Paul.

Cash Limits

The final planing method applied in the seventies was limitation of NHS budgets, in advance. Before 1976 health services were provided by the relevant Health Authorities, and paid for by the Exchequer, via the Department of Health. Negotiation between the DHSS, the Regions, and the Areas was the mechanism for controlling expenditure and keeping it within target limits. It clearly did not work; the NHS had taken 3.95% of GDP in 1949, and its share was to reach 6.1% in 1980. The Conservatives' slogan 'infinite demand, finite resources' seemed increasingly appropriate to those who could not or would not see the origins of the demands, nor the reasons for the limited resources. In an attempt to really control expenditure, the system of funding was changed. The old method had allowed a volume of services to be paid for after use. The new method paid in advance, forcing the Health Authorities to provide services within budgetary limits that were real, not targets. 'Cash-limiting', introduced in 1975-76, introduced a phase of zero growth in volume terms. Inevitably, cuts in services followed, for planned cash-limits never matched the actual costs of providing health services with this kind of planning. Only one kind of health care grew, in volume terms – private medicine.

CHAPTER 5

Going Private, Staying Public

In the late seventies the left in the labour movement became alarmed at the prospect of a two-tier health service. Private medicine had resurfaced as a political issue in 1972, when the Tory-controlled House of Commons Expenditure Committee issued a white-wash report on private practice inside the NHS. By 1976 confrontation had replaced consultation, with the BMA's consultants threatening (but never really taking) industrial action, and hospital trade unionists 'blacking' private patients in NHS pay beds.

The two-tier service had been there all along, of course. It became an issue when the 'top' tier, the private sector, became big enough to be made into political capital. The Conservatives saw the enlargement of the private sector as one element of their Long March through the institutions of the Welfare State. Labour, keen to prove its egaliatarian qualities, found in private medicine an ideal example of class privilege and corruption. Blatant enough to be obviously unpalatable to the left, private medicine (unlike private education or private housing) was small enough to be vulnerable to attack. In the end the Conservatives won the battle over private medicine, although at first glance they came off badly. A longer look at the conflict, however, suggests that the odds were stacked the Tory way all along.

Most important to the Conservatives' success was the tradition of two-tier health care. The Health Service had always been better funded and more abundant in affluent areas than in poorer ones. Teaching Hospitals, especially in London, have tended to give higher standards of care than 'ordinary' District Generals. Surgical wards have usually been better staffed, more spacious and more attractive than wards in geriatric or mental illness hospitals. Differences in quantity and quality of health service have reflected social stratification and class power in Britain. The NHS had allowed these differences to be expressed within a public institution, rather than betwen public and private institutions. The Conservative strategy aimed only at separating different levels of health care and restributing them between public and private enterprise.

Iain Macleod and Enoch Powell, both destined to become Conservative Health Ministers, wrote in a 1952 pamphlet:

> Given that redistribution is a characteristic of the social services, the general presumption must be that they will be rendered only on evidence of need, i.e. of financial inability to provide each particular service out of one's own or one's family's resources ... The question therefore which poses itself is not, 'should a means test be applied to a social service?' But 'why should any social service be provided *without* test of need?' (E Powell and I Macleod, *The Social Services – Needs and Means*, Conservative Political Centre, January 1952)

Bernard Braine, Shadow Health Minister in 1967, wrote:

> We could ensure that more is spent on medical care by introducing charges which could be covered in part ... or wholly by health insurance ... or we could encourage the growth of private medical schemes ... we might even look at the possibility of levying a hotel charge for hospital stay. (*International Medical Tribune*, October 26 1967)

Keith Joseph, reviewing the second decade of the NHS, concluded:

> The Chancellor of the day will not be willing to sign a blank cheque to the Treasury ... expenditure will have to be financed partly by contributions and partly by charges ... there may be elements in it that can be charged to patients without discouraging early treatment or unduly burdening the ill, and such charges should be subject to a means test ... contributions too can grow as average earnings grow, and perhaps they may be one day two levels of contributions: a lower one for those in a lower bracket of earnings; and a higher one for those above. (Keith Joseph *The Health Services – the Second Decade*, Conservative Political Centre, 1959)

The BMA joined in the campaign with a report on health care finance, published in 1970. In this report the BMA argued that some health services should be financed from general taxation, whilst others should be covered by separate insurance arrangements 'in which there is a direct link between the cost of supply and demand on the one hand and subscription level on the other'. And it urged that citizens should have the 'opportunity to contract out of what may be called the compulsory health insurance (that is, National Health Insurance) into an insurance scheme which offers higher benefit.' (Summary of the report *Health Service Financing,* BMA, April 1974)

The chosen mechanism for separating the different levels of medical service has been the application of budget constraints within the NHS. This limitation of the health service budget has been common to Conservative and Labour administrations, although each has its own motives for adopting the common approach.

The Conservatives' second advantage has been the dominance of medical professionals within the NHS. The medical profession, itself a tight hierarchy with hospitals specialists at its apex, mediates between the different levels of health provision, and has been allowed to equate the public good with its own interests, on the grounds that 'experts know best'. Medical professionalism has tolerated inequalities within the NHS, because those inequalities correspond to the natural, and unequal, distribution of power within medicine itself. The consultant surgeon was (and still is) more important to the general conception of health care than the doctor in the family planning clinic, or even than the consultant geriatrician or consultant psychiatrist. The dominant section of the profession directs resources into priority areas, defined on its own scale of values, whenever possible. Whether the resources are public or private hardly matters. Since the interests of the public are taken to be the interests of doctors, private medicine is good for the nation precisely because it helps its practitioners. Private medicine within the NHS was defended, in the turbulent debates of the seventies, because it drew 'excellence' (those practising privately) into the health service. The idea that money spent in Harley Street, or on NHS pay beds, might be better spent on services for the elderly, or the mentally ill, was rejected automatically – because the 'experts knew best' and therefore dominated the decision-making. The labour movement has rightly rebelled against the institutionalised privilege, without remembering its own historical acceptance of the cult of medical expertise. And the reformer's response to professional power – the evolution of a countervailing administrative force – has itself come to nothing. The new breed of administrators cannot overrule professionalism as a whole, even though they may overwhelm individual professionals. In the end, health service administration has concentrated, as it has to, on balancing the books. As budgets shrink and spending-targets are passed effortlessly, all contributions are welcome. Private finance, mediated by the busy doctors, can fill the gap.

Health as Consumption

The final Tory asset is the consumer. Wanting and needing health care, but having virtually no control over health service provision, turns the individual user of the NHS into a potential consumer. Since cash-payment has little significance within the NHS, other techniques are needed to match demand with the limited supply. The advantages here lie with the knowledgeable and educated who certainly make better use of the NHS than their less-educated peers, even though their objective need for it is probably less. If, however, the service is barely available, and a rival service exists for a fee, the user can at least pretend to be a consumer of commodities. Cash-payment even appears to equalise access to services, for access depends only on an ability to pay, and not on skill in manoeuvring through the machinery. If a skilled worker can appear to match the professional's tumble-drier, video and foreign holidays, why not also match access to the specialist, or evasion of the waiting list? In practice, of course, 'buying' health care is nothing like buying consumer goods. 'Wants' and actual needs do not correspond, expenditure cannot be predicted because needs themselves are unpredictable, and would-be consumers rarely shop around for bargains – we invariably opt for rapid solutions to worrying problems, regardless of price. That reality does not blunt consumerism, unfortunately. The idea that 'only the best will do' fits snugly alongside the belief that the 'experts know best'. Since the labour movement delegated responsibility for health care to medical professionals, and opted *against* democratic accountability within the NHS, it must bear some of the historical responsibility for the renaissance of the private medical sector.

With such advantages, why did the Conservatives take so long to win the battle over private medicine? The answer is as long as the period between the economic crises. The formation of the NHS coincided with the end of one economic crisis. The financial problems of private and charity hospitals were resolved by their nationalisation, just as they were in the mines and other basic industries. A large public sector became the skeleton of the economy; private capital was moulded in the flesh of a consumer society. Capital had no need to venture into high-risk areas, like health care. The state agreed to underwrite health service costs, and at the same time create a huge market for private commodities – the beds and syringes, and the auto-analysers, X-ray machines and drugs needed by the hospital network.

For the middle classes, the NHS was a welcome relief. They had been excluded from the panel system, and had been driven into health insurance offered by the Provident Association. By 1950 Provident Association subscriptions had fallen from a pre-war peak of nearly 10 million to a mere 120,000. Free health care, with the same doctors and the same hospitals, freed personal finance for other things. The working classes had achieved a major political objective – the extension of health services to the whole population. This was an achievement equivalent to working people getting the vote. In itself it was a break-through, and an opportunity to make further changes. Unused, it has become a symbolic monument confused with the opportunities it symbolises. At first then, only political dogmatists could complain. The natural clientele for private medicine in the early years of the NHS was the 'uppercrust', those by definition too good for a public service, and the discontented seeking further medical opinions.

Private medicine was able to survive on this client population, and slowly recruited to it, as successive governments mismanaged the expansion of the NHS. By 1960 Provident Associations' subscriptions had reached 995,000, and by 1974, over $2\frac{1}{4}$ million people were covered by private health insurance. Extra finance for private medicine was extracted from an overseas clientele, drawn principally to London's complex of Teaching Hospitals, part-time specialists and private hospitals.

yet despite the slow recovery from its post-war trough, the private sector became less rather than more significant in the provision of health care. The number of pay beds in NHS hospitals fell from 7,188 in 1956 to 5,125 in 1970, and was further reduced (through government intervention) to 2,819 by 1979. Even though the absolute number of consultants with part-time contracts (and presumably involved in private practice) increased as the NHS expanded, the proportion of the consultant workforce with part-time contracts fell from 57% in 1965 to 43% in 1976. Private practice became concentrated in particular specialist fields, especially surgery, and developed disproportionately in the affluent South East, as Table 1 shows.

The NHS Subsidises Private Medicine

The private sector's narrow base did not mean that it had no impact on the NHS. On the contrary, its concentration in certain specialities and areas focused its negative impact within the health service. Private medicine's association with the Teaching Hospitals reinforced the uneven distribution of resources already described. The powerful sections of the medical profession had little incentive to leave private practice alone, nor much enthusiasm for delegating control of decision-making to others. Taxpayers' money therefore tended to follow private money in its distribution. The private sector also harmed its neighbouring public service directly, by obtaining NHS subsidies for pay beds, and by keeping pay beds empty for potential customers whilst NHS patients were kept waiting. It was this direct injury that became a public scandal in the early seventies, and a source of open conflict after Labour's 1974 electoral successes.

The pay beds in NHS hospitals were heavily subsidised until 1976, when public outcry at the level of subsidy forced an increase in charges to private patients. In 1974 the revenue from 4,574 pay beds was £14.3 million. With running costs for beds in non-teaching hospitals standing at about £100 a week, the cost to the NHS of the pay beds was around £21 to £22 million. The shortfall of £7 million or so was due to the low rate of use of the pay beds, for only about half would be in use at any one

Table 1

Part-time Consultants by Region & Speciality, 1978

Speciality		Region	
Ophthalmology	92.2%	NW Thames	71%
General Surgery	85.6%	NE Thames	68.5%
Ear, Nose and Throat			
Surgery	84.5%	SE Thames	63.7%
Obstetrics and		SW Thames	62.7%
Gynaecology	82.4%	Merseyside	48.2%
Psychiatry	25.9%	Northern	31.1%
Mental Handicap	8.3%	Wales	37.3%
Geriatrics	6.0%	Scotland	17.8%
All specialities	47.6%	UK overall	51.8%

time. In 1971-72 private patients in pay beds were charged £1 a week to cover the capital costs of building the facility that they enjoyed; at 1971/72 prices a newly built hospital with 2,000 beds would cost about £20 million, with each bed costing £10,000. A realistic weekly rental on such a bed was estimated at the time to be about £50.

Those defending the pay beds argued that paying patients had paid their taxes and should not be surcharged for using NHS facilities, to which they had right of free access. This assumed that the practice of paying extra for preferential or special treatment was enshrined in the aims of the NHS, and therefore prefectly acceptable. Since staff and facilities were finite, such preferential treatment could only be obtained at the expense of those uanble to pay extra. The patients using pay beds to jump NHS queues, and the consultants exploiting this, were creating a two-tier health service by the back door, without public debate on the rights and wrongs of such a system. The whole purpose of the NHS was to equalise access to medical care, and those trying to buy their way round the problems of the health service, together with those profiting from the problems, were attacking the principle. In practice, private treatment put the users and the providers outside the NHS, even though they remained technically within it.

Other, hidden, subsidies came from the use of NHS time, staff and equipment for the benefit of private patients who were then not charged for what they had received. Giving evidence to the Parliamentary Select Committee on Expenditure in 1971, representatives of the Junior Hospital Doctors' Association (JHDA) alleged that:

- NHS patients needing to be nursed in single rooms were moved out to make way for private patients.
- NHS patients admitted for surgery had their operations postponed because private patients were put in at the beginning of the operation list.
- NHS patients pushed to the back of the operating list by private patients were dealt with when staff were tired and the quality of care was declining.
- Consultants 'borrowed' or even stole NHS equipment for private work.

A surgeon testifying to the same committee in 1971 explained the financial rationale for all this effort. Losing £800 a year from his NHS salary for the privlege of private practice, he operated on 6 to 8 patients privately and consulted with another 200, for which he received between £2,000 and £3,000. Inland Revenue statistics for Schedule D assessments (covering private practice earnings) in the same year showed that there were 32 medical specialists each earning £15 to £25,000 a year from private medicine, on top of their NHS salaries.

The Labour Movement's Counter Attack

The labour movement's response was to attack the pay beds within NHS hospitals. *Labour's Programme for Britain* in 1973 stated policy bluntly: 'Labour will also stop queue-jumping for hospital beds by those who can afford a private fee. Medical need shall determine the right to a hospital bed. This can only be done by the total separation of private practice from the Health Service.' The two Labour election manifestos in 1974 repeated the promise, and the National Union of Public Employees launched a campaign inside the NHS against pay beds.

A long battle between the unions on one side and a coalition of the BMA and the private sector followed, with the Labour government acting as mediator. The tactics of industrial action and public confrontation were slowly relinquished in favour of prolonged confrontation and debate between interested parties, and the government avoided taking immediate administrative action against pay beds, although it was able to do so. Instead the Labour administration chose to introduce parliamentary legislation, and committed a long period to lobbying and bargaining, during which the private sector strengthened its position. The outcome was the Health Services Board, a quango designed to phase out NHS pay beds at a rate acceptable to the private sector. It achieved a reduction in pay bed numbers, from 4,444 in 1977 to 2,819 by early 1979, but it worked under a condition entirely favourable to private medicine – no pay bed could be absorbed into the NHS unless it was replaced by a bed in a local private hospital. The Health Service Board was the first formal liaison between the private and public sectors, and was primarily concerned with maintaining a 'balance' between the two. Its creation by a Labour government demonstrates interesting, but by no means novel, features of Labour politics. Whilst hostility to private medicine was acceptable for electioneering purposes, action against pay beds was not allowed to 'get out of hand'. All political initiatives were to be confined within the mechanisms of compromise so obscure to the public and so favoured by the right. By choosing that form of politics, Labour initiated a new phase of growth in private medicine – a phase characterised by direct government support.

The Provident Association BUPA summed up Labour's role in an internal discussion paper, leaked in 1979:

> During the era of the present Labour government private practice, particularly in the independent sector, has flourished, and it is likely that if the Labour government is returned with a large majority in 1979, or even if it remains a 'hung' government, its attitude towards private practice in the coming 3-4 years will be a moderate one.

The BUPA paper went on to identify the next political tasks for the private sector:

> The Conservative Party is committed to making changes in the

private sector. Some unarguably would benefit the health insurance companies, others long term would not be in the interests of the hospital operators in the independent sector. It would appear therefore that there is a need to 'educate' Conservative politicians and broaden their philosophy so that policies will work totally to the advantage of private practice.

They were able to achieve their objective easily. But even before that happened, the labour movement had begun to make a further contribution to private sector growth.

During the late sixties and early seventies the private medical market had been unstable. Individual subscribers to health insurance had treated their policies as luxuries that could be dispensed with when personal finances were squeezed, or when private medicine was challenged politically. Overseas customers had also proved demanding and critical, and prone not to pay. A more stable 'provident population' was needed, and was found in industry. Enrolment of groups of workers, often from managerial grades, was a tradition within private health insurance. The Provident Associations worked hard to extend this tradition of group schemes to skilled, but non-managerial, employees. Their technique was to present health insurance as a valuable fringe-benefit, suitable as a bargaining counter in local negotiations, and open to use as a way round government-imposed pay restraint. The method worked, particularly where the private sector could offer convenience as a service. For example, the National Union of Seamen negotiated health insurance for oil rig workers, allowing these workers to have non-urgent medical problems resolved during their off-rig periods – a facility apparently not available through the NHS. Group enrolment became the private sector's stable base as figure 13 shows. As the private sector grew, union involvement in group insurance schemes increased despite internal union campaigns against private medicine. Of the 250,000 new subscribers recruited to private health insurance in the first three months of 1981, 30,000 came from a single agreement, between the EEPTU, the electricians' union, and the Electrical Contractors Association.

When the Conservatives won a general election in 1979, they were able to implement a long-standing Tory ambition merely by supporting changes already underway. The balance between the public and private services was already moving to the private

Figure 13
Group and Individual Enrolment to Private Health Insurance, 1966-1977

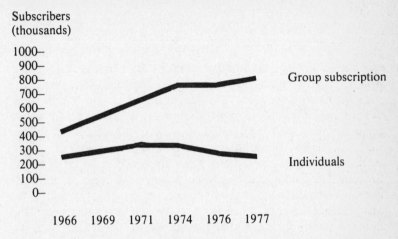

Source: Lee Donaldson Associates, *UK Private Medical Care*, 1980.

sector's advantage. Thatcher's government has accelerated, but not initiated, the shift. Against these trends, the Labour opposition is lost. It may want to abolish inequalities in health care, but it has neither the economic policy needed to finance such a reform, nor the political means to enact it. The far left repeat the slogan 'Ban private medicine', and the opportunists of Labour's right echo it. Working class organisations, in the meantime, identify their members' interests and accept the refinement of the two-tier system.

Staying Public

The sudden spate of cuts imposed by cash-limits and RAWP plans was less acceptable. The growth of the private sector had positive advantages, for some, but the restrictions on NHS budgets produced nothing but problems. The main effect was to accelerate the trend towards centralisation of services. Smaller, older hospitals were closed in favour of larger, newer (or at least refurbished) hospitals, particularly in the Regions hit hardest under the RAWP formula. Small specialist units were also merged into large, general hospitals, with the burden of closures falling on exactly those services designated for growth – mental handicap, geriatrics – or on the paediatric services, prioritised by the Court Report (1976). Convalescent and terminal care hospitals were also trimmed away in this urgent reshaping of budgets.

The logic of centralisation had largely gone unchallenged, before the rate of change became intolerable. Local communities protested, but the cult of expertise accepted by the labour movement for so long, and promoted by Labour's governments, was an overwhelming justification for change. As the cash ran out, health workers and service users began to realise the advantages of local facilities, some of which were in good condition and newly renovated, and the disadvantages of travel for both NHS staff and their patients. The fears of loss of skilled staff, as small specialist units were merged into larger District General Hospitals, and of good working relationships between health workers and their public, increased the angry reponses to accelerated closures. Job loss became an important issue, as administration demonstrated that up to 70% of their budgets went on wages and salaries, but the new awareness was too late to stop change. The NHS administration had to promote the benefits of centralisation as their need to save money became greater, and they were able to deploy logic backed by unavoidable necessity in a compelling combination.

Given the pressure for rapid change, and the administration's advantages over its opponents, the resistance was remarkably sucessful. In areas with traditions of community campaigning, and close associations between well-organised trade unionism and the community, closure plans were blocked, if only temporarily. The demonstrations, petitions, pickets, occupations and threats of strike action that brought together health workers (including professionals), trade unionists and local residents in South Wales constituted a form of public pressure that Health Authorities could not resist. Closure plans for the Amy Evans Hospital, Landsdowne long-stay Hospital, Glan Ely geriatric rehabilitation Hospital and the Prince of Wales orthopaedic Hospital at Rhydlafar, were withdrawn after public criticism and threats of industrial action, in 1978. The 'temporary' closure of the casualty department at St. David's Hospital, Cardiff, in April 1977 would have become permanent without the campaign sponsored by Cardiff Trades Council that made the Area Health Authority retreat and approach the Regional Authority for extra funds. The Cynon Valley campaign to retain

Aberdare General and Mountain Ash Hospitals and prevent transfer of services to one central site at Merthyr, in the next valley, prevented closure plans, with a community response that included local business interests as well as the labour movement, and after an eight week occupation of administrative offices in Aberdare General Hospital.

The anti-cuts campaigns in the Thames Regions were less successful, even when they used similar tactics and tried to gain wide support for their resistance. Budgets in the Thames Regions were squeezed tight under the RAWP plan, the hospital stock in London was obviously unevenly distributed and in need of rationalisation, and alternative facilities and jobs seemed available and accessible. All these factors worked to the administration's advantage, allowing campaigns (including occupations and work-ins) to be protracted, undermined, and in some cases finished by decisive intervention. The Elizabeth Garrett Anderson Women's Hospital in Central London was defended in a vigorous campaign that combined the influences of hospital staff, the women's movement, trade unions and professional workers, and forced the Health Authority to initiate further consultation. Weir Maternity Hospital was defended against closure in 1977 in a campaign that was eventually undermined by challenges to the hospital's safety record and clinical standards. Hounslow Hospital was occupied to prevent closure in October 1977, and was later emptied in the first of the hospital 'raids', its remaining 21 patients being removed in a fleet of private ambulances. The closure of Bethnal Green DGH, in East London, was proposed in 1977, despite the fact that one third of the Area's acute beds were in that hospital. Fears that the remaining facilities would be overwhelmed by the needs of people in a deprived area were not reduced by proposals to convert the hospital for use as a geriatric unit, and public campaigning forced a consultation process on the Health Authority. When the casualty department was scheduled by local supporters to keep it open, whilst workers in six other hospitals took part in protest stoppages.

Special Pleading

These campaigns were vocal, demonstrative and angry, and concentrated local grievance on tangible objectives, the bricks and mortar of threatened hospitals. Yet they rarely got beyond special pleading, arguing and pressing for their hospitals to be treated as a special case. At times that approach seemed to work very well, and when opposition was widespread and the administration's room for manoeuvre small, special pleading stopped or postponed closures. Yet the campaigns were never able to escape from the implications of their 'special case' status. If one hospital was to be reprieved, some other facility must be sacrificed to balance the books. No overall perspective existed, locally, or at any other level, to provide an alternative solution. Between the pragmatism of NHS accountants, and the revolutionary solutions of the far left, there were no answers. Inevitably, the pragmatists won the argument, particularly when they softened their blows and offered concessions. Those opposing closures often were aware of the dilemma, but unable to escape from it.

Alternative plans for the local health service were produced, with collaboration between trade unionists, professionals and community organisations, in campaigns like that of Bethnal Green, and almost certainly helped prolong the defence of threatened hospitals. Use as community hospitals was promoted by those campaigning for Hounslow Hospital, and for Willesden General Hospital (another London DGH), and their pressure put their Health Authorities onto the defensive, for a while. Those campaigns that developed comprehensive counter-proposals were able to use them, but only as far as they could penetrate the decision-making apparatus of the health service. Being out-manouevred became the normal experience for defence campaigns, and the complexity of the defence only delayed the next administrative manoeuver. When the Thornbury Annexe Children's Hospital, in Sheffield, was reprieved through public campaigning, five other hospitals were threatened with closure to permit the new Hallamshire Hospital to open. Fighting hospital closure in the late seventies was like playing Space Invaders; just as you think you have hit them all, another wave comes onto the screen.

Jobs and Service

The lack of an alternative strategy was most obvious within the trade unions. They organised some, and sometimes most, of the health workers in the threatened services, and had a line of communication to workers in the local economy through the trades councils. When the issues were clear, their organisatioon good and local support powerful, an alternative strategy could emerge and be imposed on the NHS administration. When an attempt was made to cut staffing levels at Calderstone's Hospital for the mentally handicapped, in Lancashire, the staff responded first with a work to rule, and then by occupying one block, which they ran at staffing levels that they thought desirable. Extra staff volunteered to work, beyond their normal duties, to improve patient care. The occupation – one of the first work-ins – prevented the planned staffing cuts, forced the administration to pay those who had worked, and prompted an independent inquiry that advocated increases in staffing levels.

A similar move, to close an ambulance station in Wallsend and transfer services to Newcastle, was opposed by NUPE with the threat of a work-in, and with the promise of support from local shipyards. With public pressure added, the closure plan was withdrawn, and the existing ambulance service retained. These instances were celebrated as evidence that resistance worked, and that trade union pressure alone was the essential ingredient to success. When trade unionism failed, however, as it did in the campaign to retain South London's Weir Maternity Hospital, uncritical and frustrated campaigners began to cry 'treason'. The Weir Hospital had been run down prior to closure, like so many other small units scheduled for centralisation. Its nursing staff were mostly ununionised, and were under pressure to accept relocation. The obstetric staff were doubtful, in public, about the safety of Weir Hospital, and were able to cite the high still-birth rate as evidence. The main union, NUPE, organised the ancillary staff but had little chance in an argument about clinical priorities, and understandably withdrew to a familiar issue, the defence of jobs. Once the Health Authority had pledged, and then provided, alternative employment for Weir staff, the union could only back down and call off the occupation its staff had initiated. Given the trade union movement's traditional acceptance of the cult of expertise, its failure to evolve an alternative strategy is understandable, and the climbdown at Weir was unavoidable. In the end, most of the services threatened by sudden closure or premature conversion to other uses were lost or altered because the opponents of change could not match the arguments of the NHS administration. Militancy, and the growth of widespread support for defence campaigns, depended on the strength of the alternative proposals, and not the other way round.

War of Attrition

Within the health service, the administrators had a number of advantages over their opponents. They were able to use loopholes in the regulations to accelerate change. 'Temporary' closures could be announced, without recourse to consultation through the CHCs, and quietly be made permanent, later on. Cuts in one institution could be hidden within regrading promised for another. Facilities could be run-down, by withholding repairs and staff-replacements, and by encouraging relocation of work. In the long run, the administration had power over staff, through job selection, disciplinary action, or priorities in recourse allocation. Even consultants had to accept that the administration was in charge of housekeeping, whoever really controlled the house itself, and therefore they bowed to administrative pressure for closures and changes in use. Information about services provided by the local NHS planning data and details of finance all belonged to the administrative apparatus, which could use this knowledge to present its own views as if there were no alternative. Community Health Councils could request information, but could neither control its selection and presentation by Health Authority officers, nor produce comprehensive alternative data using their own limited resources.

The administrative structure introduced in 1974 became a controlling machine by the end of the decade, incorporating NHS staff and public representatives into formal decision-making whilst imposing its own perspectives on the development of health care, according to financial criteria determined by RAWP and cash limits. This command structure, with its long-term view and its resistance to popular pressure, has been an instrument for changing the balance between public and private spending on health care. When Lambeth, Lewisham and Southwark AHA rebelled against a further round of cuts, in 1979, the Health Authority was replaced by Health Service Commissioners directly responsible to DHSS Ministers, until a new, less difficult, Authority could be assembled. After Thatcher's electoral victory, the NHS administration was encouraged to use its power against its opponents more openly and frequently, and a series of raids on hospital occupations and work-ins followed.

Defensive Tactics

The hospital work-in is an imaginative tactic that hints at workers' control, and appeals to the left. It offers a prospect of direct community influence over the local hospital or clinic, and allows the style and standard of health care to be used by the left, rather than by professionals in alliance with the right, as a positive issue. And it is very effective, in circumstances where the NHS administration has a reduced range of options whilst those opposing cuts are a cohesive force spanning service and community. It is, however, a limited defensive tactic, as the successful raids on occupied hospitals have shown. It depends on the acquiescence of the local administration, for once the local Health Authority officers feel politically free to act, the work-ins are easily broken by direct action using police, scab labour and private ambulances. The chain of raids, from Hounslow in 1977 to St. Columba's in 1982, spans the peak period of resistance to hospital closures, a transitional period between a phase of consensus management and a phase of direct rule.

Work-ins may become a useful tactic again, but not before the political balance shifts back to the centre. This may dismay some on the left, for the hospitals occupations continued the tradition of the soviets, Turin factory councils and May '68 spontaneity that is essential to one kind of socialist mythology. The attempts to set up workers' councils, new administrations for occupied hospitals, in one or two work-in's came from that tradition, revealing a narrow interpretation of 'workers' by their exclusion of professionals and their reliance solely on blue-collar workers. It does not help us much to confuse a tactic with a strategy, but it is hardly surprising, for there were no alternative views available to challenge such naive or dogmatic ideas when the cuts began to hurt. The trade unions were forced into defending the NHS, and into facing issues in health politics that were unfamiliar, and outside the scope of wage negotiation and conditions of work. The Labour Party was directly implicated in the political and ideological processes that ended in RAWP, cash-limits and service cuts, and could not help the trade union movement by intervening to defend the NHS, or even by explaining tactical options, until Labour was out of office and internal conflicts had been resolved.

If any political organisation had ever seen the NHS as an expression of continuing class conflict, during the post-war period, it had been unable to organise an appropriate response to its assessment. The assumptions about experts knowing best had influenced the political left so much that, by 1976, there was no organisation that could coordinate resistance to cuts, or provide an applicable alternative perspective for health care development. There were plenty of slogans, but they remained the abstract principles of pressure groups like the Socialist Medical Association. Even those who thought they were untainted by reformism could only respond at a local level, to local cuts.

Attempts to create a central organising force, a coordinating body, were made in these unfavourable circumstances, and like the defence campaigns themselves were more successful than their short lives suggest. The 'Fightback' group, which publicised and inspired local defence campaigns through conferences and its magazine, grew out of the Hounslow occupation and died with the 'work-in' tactic. Outside the trade union movement's official structure, suspect because of its far left tendencies, and too poor to develop beyond its original role, 'Fightback' lost its case and purpose in the administrative crackdown on Etwall pre-convalescent hospital, St. Benedict's long-stay geriatric hospital, and St. Columba's terminal care unit. It left a place for another central organiser, a new coordinating force, with a different base and a different purpose.

The new base, and the features of a second phase of campaign against NHS cuts, also appeared in the late seventies. Most anti-cuts campaigns aimed to defend existing institutions, but one very large and durable campaign defended nothing more than a plan. The town of Hemel Hempstead, in prosperous Hertfordshire, had grown so much since 1945 that it needed new health service facilities for its population of 250,000 people. A new hospital had been promised in the fifties, but had not been built by the time cash-limits were imposed on the health service.

Health Authority cuts included the planned hospital, and a local campaign – the Dacorum Hospital Campaign, named after the locality – took to the streets to demand that the promise be honoured and the planned hospital be built. The campaign was initiated by trade unionists, but not restricted to them. Local industries were involved, and suported the campaign by financing advertising, whilst factories stopped as their workforces joined demonstrations. Ten thousand people met the Labour Health Minister, Roland Moyle, when he visited Hemel Hempstead in 1977, and a torchlight procession of 5,000 presented a mass petition to Labour Secretary of State, David Ennals, when he visited the town in early 1978. Persistent pressure on the Community Health Council and the Area Health Authority, backed by another demonstration of 10,000 in the summer of 1979, forced the AHA to accept that it must apply for extra funding for the long-promised hospital. All that occurred in an area that was neither a deprived inner-city nor a traditional Labour stronghold, but an affluent town in the South East, and it defied orthodox classification. Many applauded the Dacorum's campaign's strength and style, but its significance was not realised until the second phase of resistance to cuts began, in 1982.

The London – Liverpool Axis

Cash-limits are the common background to the budgets of all NHS Regions, and create a common threat to services. Cuts imposed through application of the RAWP formula to 'overprovided' Regions discriminate against those parts of the country where private medicine is healthiest. This combination of RAWP-effects and the 'leeching' effect of the private sectors adds an extra strain to services in the South East (the four Thames Regions) and in those Regions extending roughly from London to the Mersey – the London-Liverpool axis.

These strains are compounded by the insensitivity of the planning methods used in the NHS, and their inability to cope with social factors pertinent to health care. The NHS underprovides in areas of social deprivation and consequent high need, and also in areas with expanding populations and rising demand for health services. The NHS in the inner city areas of London is underfunded, despite being in 'overprovided'

RAWP-Regions, because of social problems and their accompanying illnesses. The health service in oxford Region, on the other hand, is underfunded because a relatively more healthy population is growing faster than NHS resources. As London and other cities empty into the surrounding countryside, health services around the cities are stretched to their limits whilst the urban services take the strain of increasing unemployment and deteriorating housing.

Localised crises, like the one that developed in Oxford Region in 1982-3, are being superimposed on the general problems created by unrealistically-low cash limits. The regional variation in financial problems within the NHS corresponds to the variation in the growth, nationwide, of the private sector, and seems likely to provoke particular kinds of responses in defence of public services. The Oxford Region's Consultative Document (described in the next chapter) has been answered by a Region-wide trade union initiative aiming at co-ordinated local campaigns backed by union-sponsored alternative strategies for the Regional health services. As the financial problems accumulate and force further cutbacks in the Thames Regions, Essex, and further out along the axis, the Oxford model of opposition may become the norm, with the trade unions acting as the core of a coalition of community bodies, consumer groups and special-interest organisations concerned to defend the NHS.

Just as the balance of public and private health services will vary from Region to Region, so will the nature of health politics and resistance to cuts. This new base of opposition will need some form of national resource centre, to inform and support Regional campaigns at different levels of development. As the defence of the NHS develops regionally and locally, national coordination around new policies could become realistic and effective. Some kind of 'Health Alliance' linking service-providers and the public could emerge as the focus of health politics on a mass scale. The evolution of this kind of movement would test the left's ability to cooperate, win public support, and reject prefabricated thinking in favour of practical innovation. The changes needed in political practice are daunting: inter-union collaboration, an end of exclusiveness, and to vanguard pretensions; a new approach to the professionalism that dominates health care; and a more realistic approach to Thatcherism.

CHAPTER 6

The Mixed Economy of Health

Thatcher's government has not evolved a *new* policy for the health service. It has simply acted forcefully to resolve the economic, structural and political problems that have developed within health care in the post-war period. The Conservatives have drawn upon their fund of policies directed against the Welfare State. Once ideas about dismantling the NHS entirely were extremist expressions restricted to the far right. Now they are the subject of Cabinet discussion. Finding alternative sources of finance for the health service is, of necessity, a major concern of Thatcher's government.

The economic problems of health care are serious and uanvoidable, given the erosion of our national economy and our subordination to the EEC and America. In 1949 the NHS cost £433 million to run, taking 3.95% of the GDP and 11.8% of total public spending. By 1980 NHS expenditure had risen to £11,800 million, taking over 6% of the GDP and more than 12% of total public spending. Spending on health services has risen substantially, even allowing for inflation, whilst profit margins, output and market shares for productive industries have dropped. The trend to increase spending on health services allows only two strategic choices: either public spending on health is increased, and the economy restructured to permit this continued expenditure; or public spending is reduced because a declining national economy cannot afford it, and cannot be changed either. Not surprisingly, the Conservatives opt for the latter course. The Labour Party, the Liberals and the SDP remain unsure of which to choose, and move between the two options. Only the Communists and the far left advocate economic renewal aimed at preserving and expanding public services.

In the search for alternative methods of financing the health service the government has found a range of economic resources open to exploitation. Private capital is interested in entering the field, and takes the shape of profit-seeking hospital companies (mostly from the USA), co-operatives of doctors backed by banks, and health insurance off-shoot companies or client-organisations, plus private caterers, cleaners and laundries. From the government viewpoint the private sector contributes to health services by undertaking a range of medical and non-medical tasks, and to the national economy by reinforcing the drift toward service industries.

Community 'resources' are also plentiful, and the Tories outline their intentions for them in *Care in the Community*, a document published in 1980, in which community services were to be developed, but without any extra resources being made available for them. Local government finance can be made to cover certain kinds of services previously paid for from NHS budgets. The movement of the mentally ill or handicapped into hostels and homes supervised by social service departments, from institutions run by the NHS, shifts costs away from the health service and onto local authorities. Since local government expenditure is partially based on rates the cost is genuinely moved into 'the community'. And since cuts in central government funding of local authorities force Councils to re-assess their spending plans, the extra burden obtained from the NHS helps to sharpen councillors' minds.

Where local authority help fails, through lack of funds, then the costs and responsibilities of caring for the ill within 'the community' can be borne by family, friends and neighbours, and volunteers. A growing number of unemployed people, and particularly unemployed women, are available as unpaid labour for this work of 'community care'. The front line of health care, at least for much long-term illness and handicap, will be the social network of the ill or handicapped person. Support provided by social services department (through home helps, meals-on-wheels, social workers) will only be available to fill the gaps in the social network, as these services themselves are contracting relative to the population's needs. Medical faciltiies within 'the community' will depend increasingly on general practitioners, who have two important advantages for this government. They provide a service 'on the cheap', since they are the prototype of the contracted-out service, supplying their own premises and staff (with subsidies, of course) for the NHS.

And they are uncontrollable, with no effective mechanisms for ensuring that contracts are fulfilled and work done. Public pressure for improved general practitioner services is weakened by the difficulty in measuring the quality or quantity of services provided, or in changing them in the absence of accountability. Finally, if all other attempts to make 'the community' pay fail, charges for medical care can be considered.

Private capital appeared to be a promising source of extra money in 1979, and the government enthusiastically tried to recruit for private medicine. In June 1979 Health Secretary Gerard Vaughan wrote to reassure the BMA that the government had a wise policy towards the private sector. He anticipated collaborative development of private and public facilities at local level, and made several practical proposals to achieve this aim. Advance notification of significant new private hospitals developments, at the planning stage, was suggested as an initial phase in local consultations between private medical interests and Health Authorities. The aim of this consultation was to be orderly and effective development of private and public health services at local level – almost exactly the objective of the Health Services Board. However, instead of concentrating on a single issue – the number of beds in the private and public sectors – the new-style consultation was to work towards contractual arrangements between private and public sectors for joint provision of services, sharing of staff, collaboration in research, and shared-staff training. The Health Services Board had served its purpose as a model for this new, much-expanded, cooperation, and was abolished by the Conservatives in 1980.

Contracting Out

The Conservatives have pursued the theme of contracting-out parts of health service work to private companies. Draft circulars on the subject of contracting-out, aimed at Health Authorities, became public in the spring of 1981 and again in July 1982, but appeared to have had little impact within the NHS. In 1980 and 1981 only 0.31% of catering and 2.54% of cleaning was done privately, although a higher figure had applied to laundry services in the previous year – over 14%. In 1982 some 26 hospitals, including 9 out of 10 Army Hospitals, used private cleaners, and only 2 used private caterers. The second draft circular, leaked by the Health and Social Service Journal in July 1982, was a tetchy document acidly noting that 'Ministers have received complaints from contractors who, having submitted tenders, are kept waiting for the results.' The draft circular helpfully provided the addresses of major private contractors, but became an embarrassment to government health ministers battling hard with NHS unions over a 12% pay claim, and was withdrawn for the duration of the pay dispute. Despite the evident lack of enthusiasm within the NHS for contracting-out services, the Conservatives are able to rely on a tradition of private contributions to NHS functioning.

General practitioners have the nominal status of 'independent contractors' to the NHS, although their real situation is much more ambiguous because of huge subsidies that they receive from the state. Even so, general practice shows all the features of contracted-out services: lack of quality and quantity control over work done; variable and often poor facilities; low pay, of ancillary staff if not of general practitioners themselves; and no agreed and applied standards of training for doctors and support-staff alike. The care of the elderly infirm also relies on contracted-out services, with 30 to 40% of the 27,000 places in private nursing homes in the late seventies being occupied by patients paid for by the NHS. And contracted-out abortion services flourish, as charities are used by Health Authorities unable or unwilling to develop their own abortion facilities. It is this clinical tradition of contracting-out services that gives this government hope for further erosion of the public service. The centrally controlled structure of the NHS also offers hope to the government, for once it is fully in Conservative hands, it can be used to achieve Conservative objectives. The structural reforms of the sixties and seventies work very much in the government's favour. Once the hospital ward sister was in charge of cleaning, ward organisation and, to some extent, catering on her ward. After 1974 she had to deal with the line management of another department within the hospital – a good preparation for a future relationship with a line management outside the hospital.

The Conservatives could therefore afford to play a waiting game, although they were clearly disappointed by their lack of progress in their first two years of office. For all the tradition of contracting-out services, they also faced substantial opposition from NHS administrators, who see no financial advantage in

losing what they already had, and from trade unionists anxious
to prevent job-loss. The adminsitrators realised that to contract-
out hospital or health centre cleaning, for example, meant
retaining the in-house labour force whose wages are the major
cost of the service whilst hiring equipment and management
from an outside company. This may appeal to the workers
involved, who would retain their jobs and wages, but the
potential loss of quality-control cannot please the administrators
paying the bill. Nor can they forget that apparently cheap
outside suppliers may be operating as 'loss-leaders' to win
contracts, wipe out in-house services, and then increase charges,
from a position of strength. In the end the NHS would have to
pay bills that would cover costs, VAT on labour-costs (zero
rated in the NHS) *and* the outside company's profits.

The profit element cannot apply within the NHS, which could
only be undercut by the private sector if private suppliers were
much more efficient. If they become so much more efficient, is it
because the NHS is 'inefficient', or is it because outside
companies exclude unions and pay low wages? The economics
of contracting-out the 'hotel' services of cleaning, catering and
laundry make little sense from either management or workers
standpoints, and so prompt an unusual coalition of interest that
resists the government's plans. The Tories are understandably
annoyed by this. Conservative MP Michael Brown, described by
The Health Services newspaper as a 'director of Michael
Forsyth Associates, a public relations company which is seeking
to secure a contract with a major cleansing congolomerate', put
all his anger into a stock Tory cliché: 'it is terrible that NUPE
and COHSE should be able to hold the hospitals to ransom.
There are companies that can provide better standards of
cleansing at cheaper prices.'

Interpenetration of private and public health services requires
a healthy private sector, and this requirement has given the
Conservatives a headache. Private medicine is a fragile bloom
and contrary to its own propaganda, needs constant support.
Thatcher's government opted initially to enlarge the private
market – the insured 'provident population' – and the private
suppliers, the doctors able to see patients privately.

The Private Health Boom ... and Slump

Private health insurance was boosted in a practical way, from April 1982, by allowing tax exemption on premiums paid by employees involved in group health insurance schemes. Prior to this change, employers could claim tax exemption when they contributed to a group scheme premium, and so had a financial incentive to offer health insurance as a fringe benefit to their workers. Their employees gained the same incentive, courtesy of the government. The NHS Consultants' Contract was also modified, to abolish the difference between full-time ('whole-time') specialists working solely for the NHS and part-timers able to work in the private sector too. Now whole-time specialists can have a private practice and earn up to 10% above their NHS salary without jeopardising their salary. As confidence in the private sector's worth grew, subscriptions to health insurance increased. In 1979 private health insurance companies grew at an aggregate rate of 18%, and covered over $2\frac{3}{4}$ million people. By the end of 1980 the provident population reached just over $3\frac{1}{2}$ million, and another $\frac{1}{4}$ million were enrolled in the first three months of 1981. In 1980 the growth rate of the 'Big Three' (BUPA, PPP and WPA) taken together was 27.5%. They enthusiastically projected their growth rates to create a provident population of 12 million in 1985. A Tory miracle seemed underway.

It could not last, and even the private health isnurance companies knew it. In 1981 growth rate fell to 12%, whilst claims on insurance policies rose rapidly. Whilst the growth rate was still spectacular, it became an ominous warning for the largest health insurance company, BUPA. This organisation had expected that its new recruits would behave as others had in the past, taking an average of two years to use their private health insurance. Their claims might be bigger than any BUPA experienced since 1948, but BUPA itself would be numerically larger and well able to pay out without undue strain. Their calculation was wrong. The new breed of provident people use their health insurance soon after enrolment and juxtaposed massive claims and a reduced recruitment rate. BUPA went into the red on its current spending, and had to transfer reserves to cover the loss. As longer-term protection it restricted its clientele, increasing premiums in group schemes and limited the services available under the insurance policies by declaring certain highly-expensive private hospitals 'out of bounds'. The hospitals were mostly American-owned, and profit seeking. Whilst the US-controlled hospitals protested their innocence, they got the message and realised that private medicine in Britain was not the wide-open market that they had entered in 1979 and 1980. Nor did the other health insurance companies miss the point, as high-spending refugees from BUPA's premium-hike transferred allegiances. The Tory honeymoon for private medicine ended in 1982.

The bubble burst for the private hospitals too. Fifty-three new private hospitals were planned for 1981, but only 11 new plans were notified in the twelve months prior to October 1982. Even when the Government was enthusiastic to sell off public facilities (like St Columba's Hospice for the dying, on a prime site in North London) buyers were nervous. Capital follows confidence and confidence has never been very strong when it came to building new hospitals or even to converting existing ones. Public announcements of new private hospitals developments have tended to provoke protests, and nothing un-nerves financial backers more than picket lines and a bad press. They rightly worry at the prospect of delayed completions because of industrial action, of prolonged battles with planning committees, of rising interest charges on capital loans, and of nervous clients unsure of entering their political dispute by walking through a new hospital's gates. The Conservative government did what it could to reduce the private sector's anxiety. Control over private sector developments was transferred from the Health Services Board to the Secretary of State for Health. Restriction on bed numbers in new hospitals were eased, so that private developments could be larger than before without needing special authorisation. Conversely, opponents of any new private venture were required to demonstrate that the new development 'adversely affects' the NHS – a difficult task when the government sees private capital as a saviour of health care!

It did not help. By mid-1982 the government's tactic of encouraging the private sector and constraining the public service had reached its limits. Spending on the NHS continued to rise, although inflation meant that it bought fewer and fewer services. The private sector was suffering serious growing pains, despite much pampering. The only options left for a government committed to the reconstruction of the national economy at the expense of the public sector (and the public generally), was to dismantle the NHS in part or whole. This became a preoccupation and the cause of much embarrassment for the government in the last few months of that year.

Two Tory Options

Tory policy options became public at the September 1982 Party Conference. The far-right leaked a 'Think Tank' discussion Paper aiming at ther replacement of the NHS by a wholly insurance-based service. Immediately afterwards Oxford Regional Health Authority Officers, after consultation with the Labour RHA Chaiman, launched a Consultation Document detailing massive service cuts within their Region. Conservatives demonstrated their lack of self-confidence, even after the public response to the Falkland adventure, by promptly disowning each option. Margaret Thatcher announced that the NHS was 'safe' with the Conservatives, although she managed to add 'however financed'. Tory collusion in the proposals outlined by the Oxford RHA Paper was hotly denied, even though Under Secretary for Health Geoffrey Finsberg had written to Oxford RHA in the Summer, urging them to take 'painful decisions' to stay within their budget. And the Think Tank report was shelved, despite rumour that it had the support, within Cabinet, of Keith Joseph and Thatcher herself.

Despite these denials, the options remain valid. The logic of Conservative policy forces the government into increasingly radical action, since economic recovery will not come to its aid. The *choice* of option is the Tories' current political problem, and it was this that threatended to divide the Conservative Party just before a general election. In balance, the Tories seemed likely to opt for the Oxford approach now, whilst keeping the Think Tank plan in reserve for a second term of office. This solution has many advantages. The Oxford plan appears to be simple obedience to economic necessity, enacted by a Health Authority and not by the government itself. It preserves a large part of the NHS, whilst forcing (rather than encouraging) the private sector to expand. And it can be carried out Region by Region with a flexible timetable, even if the Conservatives lose a general election because their economic policies fail. The Think Tank report, on the other hand, could have provoked a pre-election debate on the virtues and vices of Welfare and a public service – a debate that the Tories doubt they could win. Only a party fighting an 'all-or-nothing' campaign would lead with such a policy. Much better to re-introduce the idea after the Conservative majority in the House of Commons has been enlarged, and their economic policy endorsed (for whatever reasons) by the electorate.

The Oxford Region's proposals are, therefore, the shape of things to come. Oxford Region, covering the four counties of Northamptonshire, Buckinghamshire, Oxforshire and Berkshire, is especially vulnerable to cash-limits. Its population growth has exceeded the estimates made using the clumsy RAWP formula, whilst its pioneering role in economic use of facilities has left little fat on the bone to trim away. The solutions to ever-tighter budgets have been to postpone, and then abandon, all plans for expanding the health services within the Region. When planning for zero-growth, despite a growing and ageing population, seemed insufficient to stay within cash-limits, Regional Officers assembled a packet of possible service cuts. They included:

1. a residence qualification, requiring people to have lived with the Region for an unspecified time period before they were eligible for NHS treatment within the Region. This idea effectively revived the Elizabethan Poor Law provision for returning the needy to their parish of origin;

2. closure of casualty departments at weekends, or restriction of casualty services to nine departments in the four counties, plus provision for charging accident victims;

3. closure of wards, or whole hospitals if possible, with most surgery being done on a day-care basis from outpatients clinics. Most NHS posts would be converted into part-time jobs;

4. a reduction in maternity inpatient care to 24 hours after confinement;

5. the closure of mental handicap and mental illness hospitals, without waiting for local authorities to make alternative provision for those living in them;

6. transfer of non-urgent surgery and family planning services to the private sector;

7. either the introduction of charges to patients for NHS transport, catering and laundry, or the use of volunteers to run these services without charges;

The Oxford approach is very important to the Conservatives. Not only does it represent a 'softly, softly' option, compared with the Think Tank proposals. It also elaborates earlier Conservative policies, particularly on charges, residence qualifications and contracting-out *medical* services. As well as showing the other hard-pressed Regions a way round their difficulties, it also offers an escape-route through 'special case' status for Oxford Region, should the going become rough.

The Oxford proposals roll together individual Tory policies and aply them in a new way. Charges for care of accident victims, for example, were selected by the Thatcher government as an objective early in its term of office, but were rejected because the motor insurance companies which would have paid for the medical treatment were unenthusiastic. Oxford Region's plan changed the idea of such a charge from an option to a necessity. The same applies to charges for catering, laundry and transport, which have been in the Tory armoury since the NHS was founded. Residence qualifications are newer, but also came into force in 1982 for those defined as 'not normally resident' in the UK. From 1 October 1982 anyone judged to be ineligible for free hospital treatment because they were 'not normally resident' could be changed (except in emergencies and for infectious diseases) for their medical care. A pilot study had demonstrated that this qualification applies to only 0.5% of the people using NHS hospitals, and probably cost more to apply than it saved. The government however favoured its introduction for a variety of reasons.

The residence qualification helps create a climate in which charges for medical care become acceptable, and, like all charges, also helps to establish the idea of *eligibility* for free health care, in place of the idea that services are freely available at the time of need. It also creates and tests the mechanisms for charging patients that would be needed if the NHS were replaced by an insurance-based health service. And it immediately deflects some people into the private sector, where they can avoid confrontations and challenges over their eligibility to NHS treatment. Finally, Oxford Region's proposal to hand over non-urgent surgery and family planning to the private sector came as a welcome relief to government and private medicine alike. Again, necessity appears to replace choice in opting for private solutions to public sector problems.

Necessity, however, is in the eye of the beholder. The Conservatives move from choice to necessity in their attitude towards private penetration of the NHS in 1982, but their opponents did not. The government's second priority, after elaborating its policy on a public-private mix for health, has been to demolish opposition inside and outside the NHS. It has pursued this objective in the same way that it elaborated its policy, along many lines. A further administrative reform in 1982 was intended to streamline the control structure purged of hostile lay officials – particularly the key Health Authority chair posts held by Labour Party members or sympathisers. Community Health Councils were singled out for attack, and the trade unions within the NHS became a priority candidate for both harassing actions and direct confrontation.

Patients First?

Structural reform was an easy option for the new government in 1979. The apparatus created in 1974 seemed to satisfy no-one, and was criticised for being cumbersome and bureaucratic, with slow decision-making and poor communication between its three tiers. In 1977 the DHSS had admitted to the House of Commons Public Accounts Committee that there had been an increase of 16,400 administrators and clerical workers after 1974, and this fuelled charges of 'bureaucracy' even though some of these staff had been transferred from local authority health services, or had been recruited for the new Community Health Councils. The 1974 reorganisation had proved very costly in both financial and moral terms, and inevitably became the subject of study by the Royal Commission on the NHS (1976-79). The Royal Commission advocated that one administrative tier below Region should be abolished, that CHCs should be strengthened in their 'watch-dog' role, and that the functions of Family Practitioner Committees (FPCs) should be incorporated into the main administrative structure of the health service. The Conservatives accepted only the first proposal.

The government's consultative document *Patients First*, published at the end of 1979, in effect advocated the abolition of Area Health Authorities, reaffirmed the independence of FPCs, and flew a kite about the continued usefulness of the

Community Health Councils. Below Regional level revamped DHAs were to run the service, with an increased professional input to decision-making, and reduced trade union influence in policy making. With the DHAs the emphasis was to be placed on units of management, whether an individual hospital or a District Service like psychiatry, at the expense of forward planning and cross-disciplinary coordination. New boundaries for DHAs reduced their overlap with local government, but match the public sector much more closely to the growing private hospital network. Under the banner of devolution of responsibility, the Conservatives aimed to weld efficient management to professional dominance in a way that previous governments had not thought desirable. The Tories reaffirmed that clinical effectiveness could and should be left to the professionals, and that managerial efficiency would make 'good medicine' possible. The model for the new, streamlined service was precisely the idealised private hospital that the Conservatives favoured. The public bring the problems, the professionals solve them, and administrators safeguard the cash flow. All ideas of preventive care, of assessing and meeting people's needs (as distinct from their wants), and of services for whole populations, are subordinate to the doctor, his patient, and the illness.

The first obstacle tackled by Thatcher's government was the potential opposition role of the Community Health Councils. In *Patients First* their value as watch-dogs was questioned, their cost (only £4 million a year) underlined, and their continuation under the new system challenged. The hostile response to this indirect attack on CHCs included criticism from general practitioners, and checked the government. When the broad outlines of *Patients First* were endorsed, in 1980, the Community Health Councils were reprieved, subject to further review. That review came in 1981 with a consultative paper devoted to the size, scope and activities of the CHCs. Mild in tone, this government plan advocated smaller Health Councils, with a reduction in local government and trade union representation on them. They would be restricted to dealing with purely local issues, and would be heavily influenced by voluntary organisations, themselves susceptible to Conservative control. Whilst the government's attack on the CHCs is a small campaign in the overall war, it has had its impact, allowing

Health Authorities to publicly attack CHCs openly resisting cuts or promoting national policy issues.

Another round of reorganisation, and a fencing match with the Community Health Councils, could neither make nor break the momentum of change initiated by the Conservatives. For the government the decisive battle in the NHS could only be fought with the trade union movement. The major obstacle to privatisation of non-medical services within the NHS was, and still is, the public sector unions. And the major obstacle to the development of private medicine at the expense of the NHS is the wider trade union movement, and the impact it could have, directly and through the Labour Party, on the electorate in the key marginal constituencies that the Conservatives must continue to hold to win elections.

The first attack on NHS unions was targeted on types of industrial action involving breach of contract rather than withdrawal of labour. This kind of action, taking the form of go-slow, work-to-rule, overtime-ban or provision of emergency services only, had predominated over full strike action in all NHS disputes, and was a logical choice for the government. In a circular called *If Industrial Relations Break Down* (HC-79-20), issued in the winter of 1979, the government advised NHS managers on the range of sanctions against individual workers that were open to them, should disputes arise. Union protest against the circular highlighted its recommendations for withholding pay from staff providing less than normal services, and paying those who crossed picket-lines, but the circular was not withdrawn. Equally ominous were proposals that Health Authorities could prepare in advance for disputes by organising volunteers and arranging alternative services, like catering, laundry or telephone communications, should normal services be withdrawn.

The Conservatives want to give local NHS managers more autonomy for dealing with disputes, whilst creating a climate of fear amongst employees. The importance of the circular was that it implied that NHS managers would inflict sanctions on individual workers rather than take legal action against their unions. This threat fitted a longer-term strategy of undermining unionism, for it demonstrated that the unions did *not* act as a shield between employee and manager. In practice, the autonomy of local managers was to be more apparent than real.

The next major dispute, in 1982, demonstrated how little power to settle disputes lay at local level, and revealed the unimportance of purely local conflicts. Where local autonomy was enlarged, it was used by NHS administrators to break resistance to cuts, as in the notorious 'raids' on occupied hospitals like those at Hounslow and St Columba's in London.

The 1982 Pay Dispute

Having drawn limits around the favoured tactics of NHS unions, the Conservatives tried to cut off outside support through legal restrictions solidarity action and public picketting, in the Employment Act (1980). With their legal weapons deployed, they then provoked a set-piece battle over a 12% pay claim, in the spring of 1982.

The claim for a 12% increase for all NHS workers was presented in a joint demand by unions that had united, for the first time, on a pay issue. The TUC's Health Services Committee, previously dismissed as a deadlocked body overshadowed by inter-union rivalries, became a coordinated leadership for the joint campaign. Professional organisations, like the Royal College of Nursing and the Royal College of Midwives, were drawn into the wake of the trade union initiative, because their own membership responded enthusiastically to the 12% demand, even though they would not accept some trade union tactics.

The campaign for a 12% increase was based solely on maintaining the real value of earnings in 1982. It could not be, and was not intended to be, an escape from low pay status. One estimate suggested that 40% of a million-strong NHS workforce received a basic wage so low that they qualified for Family Income Supplement, and were therefore on or close to the poverty line. Table 2 shows how gross incomes compared, across the workforce.

The real situation was worse than these pay levels suggest. Health workers boost their incomes through abnormally high levels of overtime and shift work. If these payments are excluded, the average weekly wage of women in nursing fell from £3 per week *above* the average for all non-manual women workers to £3.90p per week *below* the average. Women ancilliary workers suffered a similar fall, from £1.30p per week *above* the average manual wage to £3.40p per week *below* it. Overtime and shift work payments had become so important because inflation had eroded the basic wage for several years; between 1980 and the beginning of 1982 NHS workers had experienced a 9% fall in their standards of living. In addition charges for the board and lodging of live-in nurses were due to rise by between 18% and 33% in 1982, and an increase in the employee's National Insurance Contribution was also scheduled. For nurses the erosion of real earnings stretch back to the Halsbury Report, with a drop of 3.5% in real terms in nurses' salaries between 1975 and 1981, whilst other workers had registered a rise of 3.1% during the same time.

Table 2
Average Gross Weekly Earnings For Full Time Staff, 1981

	Male £	Female £
all non-manual, UK	163.1	96.70
NHS admin & clerical	155.30	88.50
all workers, UK	140.50	91.40
NHS ambulance staff	128.40	-
NHS nurses	127.40	99.70
NHS maintenance	126.50	-
all manual	121.90	74.50
NHS ancillary staff	99.30	75.80

Source: New Earnings Survey, 1981.

The government's insistence that it could only offer a 4% increase was bound to trigger a pay campaign. The opening skirmish, with 4,000 nurses demonstrating in London against the 4% limit, was followed by a period of sabre-rattling. Hoping to divide unionists from professionals, the government announced an extra 2.4% for nurses and 'para medical' workers (physiotherapists, radiographers and other technical staff) in early March. They were answered by a one hour stoppage in mid-April, then a two hour stoppage and ban on non-urgent admissions (initiated by COHSE) at the end of the month. Trade union activists were pessimistic about the responsiveness of health workers, and unused to trade union unity within the health service. Yet in early May NUPE branches voted overwhelmingly against the government's modifed offer, and the first one day strike, on 19 May, was bigger than expected. Miners in four Yorkshire pits walked out of their workplaces in support of the NHS claim, openly challenging the government's recent employment legislation.

The first all-union two hour stoppage occurred on 27 May, and the government called on Health Authorities to stand firm on the government line. The second Day of Action, on 4 June, coincided with the RCN's rejection of the modified pay offer by a vote of 2 to 1 in a secret ballot of membership. The government were clearly alarmed, and escalated the dispute by putting troops and police on standby for the third one day strike, on 8 June. Yorkshire and Nottinghamshire miners joined in the dispute, together with the other public sector workers. On 9 June the government restated its position, refusing to grant 'new money' to meet the health workers' claim, and was criticised for its intransigence by the Health Authorities Conference on 11 June. The Conservative position had become untenable. Their Employment legislation seemed inoperable, giving the breadth of support for the NHS workers in other industries, whilst the health service managements could not or would not act as government buffers. The response to the Wales TUC's one day strike on 16 June punched the message home. Every mine in South Wales shut down, the hospital service was paralysed, and 20,000 marched through Cardiff in support of the 12% claim. By the next day 700 of the nation's hospitals have been reduced to emergency services only.

To pre-empt a national TUC one day strike called for 23 June, the government made a second pay offer on 21 June, within the range of $5\frac{1}{2}$ to 7%, and modified it again the next day to between 6 and $7\frac{1}{2}$%. It did not stop the TUC day of action affecting 1,800 hospitals and involving both public and private sector workers. Trade unionists remained surprised at the speed with which the dispute escalated, but went on to organise for a three day strike between 19 July and 21 July, and a five day strike later in the summer. The government hit back by purging the Regional Health Authorities of chairmen hostile to the government's attitude, and stood fast.

The growing trade union militancy, bolstered by another

rejection of the government's pay offer by the RCN membership focussed on the next national day of action called by the TUC, on 22nd September. The day seemed to have been a devastating blow to the government. A huge demonstration of 120,000 people streamed through London, and smaller marches wound through at least fifty other cities and towns. Millions of workers from private and public sector industries took part in action of one kind or another, from token one hour stoppages to picketing hospitals. Despite government claims to the contrary, every major industry was involved in one way or another, and once again the government's law on solidarity action was shown to be ineffective. At that point, with thousands on the streets and donations pouring into strike funds, the campaign faltered.

The government refused to move, and the trade unions had run out of ideas. The pessimists and the right within the trade union movement had misjudged the responsiveness of health workers in the early stages of the campaign, and they could now reasonably argue that the seven month battle was wearing trade unionists down and making victory less and less possible. Anyway, the government had made three new offers since March, and was hardly likely to give in any further and risk a major breach in its public sector pay-policy. The optimists, and the far left, saw the dispute in simple industrial terms. If the bosses would not cough up, shut down the factories! Indefinite industrial action, without emergency cover (in breach of the TUC code) would effectively close the NHS and bring the issue to a head. When confronted with the problem that shutting down the hospital service would hit the working class, not the bosses, some argued that such a blow would wake up the working class and set it marching on Whitehall.

Between these two options those trying to preserve both trade union unity and militancy struggled to find new tactics, and more weak points in the government's defences. In the event they failed, but not for lack of effort. The rolling programme of regional action days, scheduled from 4 to 20 October, was designed to demonstrate to the broader labour movement that NHS workers did have industrial muscle, and were prepared to use it. The regional actions were hastily organised by weary activists within a workforce that sensed that it could no longer succeed. Local action could not influence the government after it had survived the massive display of trade union force on 22

September, and health workers knew it. Professional organisations began individual talks with the DHSS, and the united campaign broke up. By December a compromise had been reached, giving differential awards to professionals and non-professionals, and stretching a 12% offer over nearly two years, not one.

The health workers could have won their claim outright, but it would have required a political intervention, not an industrial one, to break the Conservatives' resolve. Had the Labour opposition entered the conflict immediately after 22 September, using the 12% claim as an introduction to a much broader issue – the defence of the NHS – the government would have had much less room to manoeuvre. The trade union movement threatened to break the government's pay-policy, and had violated its Employment Act, but the Conservatives could survive such reverses. A Labour campaign for the NHS, coming just as the Think Tank report and the Oxford Region document hit the headlines, would have been a much more serious threat. Conservative ambitions then required another term of office, and a bigger majority. Health cuts were imminent in areas of the South East of England which the Tories had won by small margins in 1979. New populations in New Towns had to fight for services that were taken for granted, or even over-abundant, in older towns and cities. Conservative voters might desert to the Liberal-SDP Alliance, or even to Labour, if *their* health services fail to materialise or to function properly. The last thing Thatcher's Cabinet could afford before a crucial election was a public conflict over the *principles* of the NHS. Rising unemployment for some could, perhaps, be offset by falling mortgage repayments for others, and a little patriotism could cover many sins. But nothing known to Conservatism (apart from another war) could save them if Labour succeeded in branding them as the 'destroyers of the NHS'.

Sadly, the Labour Party did not take this opportunity to attack. It was not for lack of commitment, witnessed by the immense work done by Labour Party activists and by the presence of MPs and Councillors on demonstrations and public platforms. Nor was it solely because so many in the Labour Party were playing 'hunt the Trotskyist' through the party apparatus. It was because the Labour Party was no longer sure that it had the answers to the problems of the NHS. How could it be confident, after the last Labour government had engineered a major boost for private medicine and confronted low-paid workers in the health service with pay restraint? 'Realism' and determination still belonged to the Conservatives, and they exploited their advantage. The defeat of the health service workers has broken the stalemate the Tories faced at the beginning of 1982. Unionists are demoralised and demobilised, and divided from professional workers. Their resistance to cuts and privatisation has been weakened. Their numbers will be reduced as health workers defect to professional organisations that are so open to Conservative influence. The Conservatives have ensured that they will dominate the politics of health in the 1980s regardless of whether they win general elections.

CHAPTER 7

Commerce and Professionalism

The Tories have established the rules for health politics in the 1980s. They have given an impetus to private medicine, and emphasised the belief that medicine should respond to wants more than to needs. They have initiated structural change in NHS administration to favour a 'mixed economy of health', and they have weakened trade unionism and strengthened professional organisations.

If the Labour Party remains true to form, it will react to the growth of private medicine, and to the structural reforms that promote the mixed economy of health, with strong countervailing policies. Should Labour win a general election during the 1980s, its government may or may not implement these policies, but it will be under pressure to do so from within the party and the trades union movement. Labour will *not* evolve a new approach to the rivalry between trade unions and professional organisations, unless it breaks with its traditions. A tacit agreement between Labour and the BMA permitted the NHS to be established with minimal conflict, and no doubt was a necessary and expedient compromise. It shaped health politics for thirty years, until the Thatcherite breakthrough in 1979, and disarmed the left by surrendering control of the professions to Conservatism. Labour retreated into its 'safe areas', the trade unions, whilst Conservatism re-captured the professional bodies that defined the nature of 'public service'. An understanding of professionalism, and its relationship to unionism, is still missing from Labour thinking. Without that understanding, Labour's chances of once again controlling the development of health services seem small.

The Professionals

Professionalism within health care is based on the idea of

'service' and on the practice of trade. It is a market concept, expressed in the relationships between a customer (the patient), a tradesman (the professional) and assorted suppliers (the drugs industry, other superior professionals). 'Trade secrets' are necessary for the maintenance of the market relationship, and permit professionals to define themselves as special, and beyond the control of those ignorant of these 'trade secrets'. The 'autonomy' of health professionals – particularly doctors – rests on the range of their trade secrets. When nursing is restricted to mopping-up vomit, emptying bedpans and washing the bed-bound, it is only a special example of the caring role usually allotted to women, and nurses are therefore allotted the same autonomy as women generally. Nursing 'professionalism', therefore, aims at acquiring trade secrets (more politely called professional skills and knowledge) to give some nurses more autonomy, status and money. The evolution of special skills and knowledge necessitates a special education, with access to it restricted to ensure that the market is not overloaded with tradesman.

Once acquired, the trade secrets justify special rewards and privileges. One of these rewards is access to the special education needed for the trade, allowing professionalism to be kept within the family. The market has been largely abolished in health care in Britain, yet market relationships determine how health professionals work. The medical profession is the most evolved professional group, and has resisted change in its status and role whilst retaining close contact with a residual real market, in private practice. Private practice may be marginal to health care, but it is central to medicine, for it is the purest expression of medical professionalism. Other health professions either shape themselves on the medical template, and evolve market relationships before finding a market, or attempt a redefine professionalism, without the market.

This latter option is open, within professionalism, and even within medicine. The Labour government of 1945-50 may have relegated its own experts, the SMA and the MPU, to the sidelines, but it did abolish the market from health care for almost the whole population. Private medicine remains a secondary factor in health service provision, despite the boost it has received from the Conservatives, and is likely to remain so unless the far right achieves its ambition and replaces the NHS with an insurance-based system. Professionalism based on concepts and practices unrelated to market mechanisms remains both possible and necessary whilst a public sector survives within health care. The political significance of professionalism, therefore, is not simply that it reflects the realities of the market economy, but that it continually experiences an internal conflict between its market origins and its current dependence on public funds.

The conflict acts as a force for change within organisations like the BMA and the RCN, but it is not the most significant such force. The market itself dominates change within professionalism, reorganising it according to technological development and the sexual and racial divisions of labour. Within medicine technological advances in surgery have re-ordered the professional hierarchy. Before the NHS surgery was a field open to general practitioners, working in cottage hospitals, with very variable results in terms of the quality and quantity of operations performed. The NHS allowed hospital specialists to exclude GPs from surgery, and to develop its technical content until the transplantation of organs, the reconstruction of arteries in the heart or limbs, and the repair of massively injured bodies, became possible. Orthopaedic surgeons were a 'progressive' group before the Second World War, for they had low status and poor facilities, and faced a huge amount of unmet need. The NHS transformed their work and changed their position, by promoting the development of their technical craft until artificial hip joints became commonplace, accident surgery routine and surgery to the spine possible and worthwhile. Now the orthopaedic surgeons lead the private medical field and are in the front ranks of the profession. Their 'progressive' role has been taken up by other low-status, underfunded disciplines, like psychiatry, general practice and geriatric medicine, where scope for private practice is limited. It is these disciplines that act as the 'natural' homes for women doctors and overseas medical graduates.

Within nusing similar changes occurred. The NHS created a new category of nurse, the State Enrolled Nurse (SEN), to allow faster expansion in hospital staffing, and also recruited more untrained nursing auxiliaries. Freed from some tasks, the more qualified State Registered Nurses evolved new specialised roles in surgical wards, and in intensive care, coronary care and premature baby units. The new stratum of technical nurse-specialists evolved just as the middle-class Matrons were replaced by a career-structure of nurse-managers. This twin birth allowed a fuller expression of the sexual division of labour within nursing. Rational, business-like men rose through the managerial career structure and obtained salaries appropriate to family breadwinners; caring, but skilled, women filled the technical roles in the new specialisms. Immigrant workers, from Ireland, Africa, the West Indies, Malaysia and the Philippines mostly took the SEN and nursing-auxiliary jobs, forming the semiskilled and unskilled workforce in Britain's NHS, just as their contemporaries formed the same workforce in South Africa, Australia and US industries.

Technological development reorganises the relationships between professions as well as within them. The progress made in investigative techniques since 1948 created a new profession of medical laboratory technologists. These technicians became highly skilled, and their technology was labour-intensive. Measurement of chemical levels in blood, urine and other body fluids was a technician's skilled task, as was the preparation for microscopic examination of blood samples or body tissues. Technological change has automated their work-processes, so that a single machine can measure the levels of several different chemicals simultaneously in a rapid sequence of different samples. Routine blood analysis, and mechanised preparation of materials, mean that only the special cases need individual attention, which increasingly comes from the medically-qualified pathologist rather than the more narrowly-trained technician. Laboratory technicians are slowly evolving into machine-minders, whilst pathologists take over the skilled tasks.

Medicine in the Market Place

The conflict between the mercantile past and the public sector present is a second force for change with the professions. The virtual abolition of financial worries about health care means that the evolving health sciences can be at the service of the whole population. If some have better access, and get better care, than others, we can legitimately ask health professionals why they do not practice what they preach about 'service'. And if health sciences have developed enough to prevent ill health, we can also legitimately ask professionals why they do not use that preventive science, but rather concentrate on attempting to cure established disease. They have many answers to the questions. Some would emphasise the historical legacy of curative medicine, and the difficulties always faced by those trying to change traditional ways of doing and thinking. Others would blame the victims of disease for their bad habits, slow understanding and delayed requests for medical help. All would describe one detail of the main problem, in the hopes of concealing its overall character. Just as abortion would be a sacrament if men became pregnant, so health professionals would stampede into preventive work, if prevention could be made into a marketable commodity. The underlying conflict for health professionals, and particularly for doctors, is between the possibilities derived from evolving sciences, and the market relationships that determine health care provision. This confict could transform and redefine professionalism, if not resolved, however inadequately or temporarily, through the political action of professional organisations allied to capital. This, then, is the challenge of professionalism to the left in the eighties. Can the conflict between science and practice be resolved in a different way, through the creation of a new professionalism?

Medicine's market-place origins shine through in every area of clinical activity, from the most dramatic open-heart operation to the briefest consultation in a lock-up surgery. The NHS has community, specialist and super-specialist services derived from a military model, perfected in the First World War, when frontline casualty stations sorted out the injured into those treatable on the spot, those needing treatment in hospitals at the rear, and those beyond hope of recovery. General practitioners deal with what they can, pass to the hospital specialists the problems that are beyond the scope of GP treatment, and deflect those whose problems are judged to be non-medical.

The modern system differs from the military model in only one respect; little effort is made to find the 'casualties', who are expected to present themselves to their general practitioners, in one way or another. This orientation to demand, not need, is characteristic of almost all medicine, and reflects the customer-tradesman relationship. The military model, on the other hand, depended upon assessments of 'need', which over-rode the wants of individual injured soldiers in a way that would be unacceptable to health professionals and public alike within a market economy. If the military system became overloaded by excessive casualties, so that hospitals were filled, medical supplies used up, and nurses and surgeons exhausted, more and more injured men became hopeless cases, simply for lack of resources.

In a peace-time context, if the community services seem in danger of being overwhelmed by either demand or need, resources are restricted to a portion of the population. Before the creation of the NHS access to medical care was restricted by financial barriers, and through the unequal distribution of medical resources. The NHS lifted the financial barriers, and successfully redistributed resources, up to a point. The medical profession then created new barriers, particularly within the frontline of general practice. People want easy and rapid access to an individual doctor with whom they have an established relationship. Lifting the financial barrier uncovers the previously hidden demand and need for medical attention, particularly amongst the poorest and least healthy people. One response to increased demand and need is to increase supply, by increasing the number of general practitioners, particularly in the most needy areas – the working class areas within and around cities and conurbations. The alternative is to rebuild the barriers between general practitioners and their patients, by grouping practices and increasing the distance between doctor and patient, by introducing appointment systems, by using deputising services for house calls at night and weekends, and by delegating first-contact to receptionists or nurses. Both responses have occurred, but the latter dominates.

GPs – Surplus and Shortage

The number of general practitioners increased from 18,615 in 1948 to 27,700 in 1977. This compares with an increase from 13,100 hospital doctors in 1948 to 39,500 whole-time equivalent doctors employed by Health Authorities in 1977. GP numbers have increased by half, whilst hospital doctors have nearly trebled in strength. The redistribution of general practitioners occurred alongside the redistribution of hospital services, but again failed to match it in scope. The increased number of doctors trained during and after the 1939-45 war produced a medical glut in the early years of the NHS, and young doctors were forced into the only vacancies available in industrial areas. They took some of the new medical sciences with them, and made a big difference to standards of care, but there is little reason to believe that they did so out of choice. By 1956 this redistribution according to principles of supply and demand had ceased, and by 1961 it had gone into reverse. Between 1961 and 1967 the proportion of the population in England and Wales that lived in areas defined as 'under-doctored' rose from 17% to 34%, and GP vacancies in industrial areas became open to immigrant labour. Of the 169 new general practitioners who began work in under-doctored areas between October 1968 and October 1969, 164 came from abroad.

The situation was changed in post by the 1966 GP Charter, which subsidised general practice and provided the resources for renewal that independent contractors could not find for themselves. Local authorities in industrial areas realised that they faced serious shortages in GP numbers in the seventies, and took advantage of urban redevelopment programmes to replace old lock-up, shop-front surgeries with purpose-built health centres on housing estates. With better facilities available, another generation of doctors moved into general practice in industrial areas, giving the cycle of redistribution its first truly planned turn.

The reconstruction of barriers proceded at a faster pace. One study of urban general practice found that the proportion of the population with GPs operating appointment systems had risen from 15% in 1964 to 75% in 1977. Yet waiting time for patients in the surgery had not been reduced significantly by the appointment system, and 30% of those questioned reported that they could not get appointments on the same day. The delay in getting appointments acted as a deterrent to consultation for 8% of those who had to wait until the next day, and for 40% of those who had to wait three days or more. The extent of the delay was not related to the size of a group general practice, but it was longer for doctors who worked from health centres. In 1964, 9% of GPs used a commercially-organised deputising service (of on-call doctors) for night calls. This proportion had risen to 26% as regular users and 18% as occasional users of such services, by 1977. Daytime house calls shrank from 22% of all consultations in 1964 to 13% in 1977, whilst overall consultation rates remained steady, or only increased slightly. Significantly, 60% of the general practitioners studied thought that the number of consultations per patient had risen, although there was little objective evidence of this. This reorganisation within general practice also followed the semi-nationalisation of 1966, with its provision for extra staff and its inducements for group work. It has meant that individual patients are less likely to see their doctors on the same day, less likely to be seen by them at home, and less likely to be attended by them or their partners in an emergency.

Whether this made any real difference to the quality of medical care is difficult to tell, since medical professionals do not readily permit outsiders to measure the quantity or quality of the service that they provide, and are equally slow to assess their own work. Consultations have been delayed, the consultation rate held more-or-less steady, and out-of-hours work devolved or simply discontinued. The net result certainly favours the GP, who deals with a similar workload in a more orderly way, within more normal hours, whilst using better facilities and earning more money. Where financial barriers once organised demand, administrative barriers now operate.

Pathology and Progress

This evolution in the market relationship between general practitioner and patient has occurred concurrently with changes in patterns of disease, and with actual and potential developments in medical science. The GP no longer watches in each consultation with a child for the signs of polio, nor prepares for home confinements, nor sifts through the daily cases of winter bronchitis for the weekly find of pneumonia. Since infectious diseases have declined, their place must be taken by new problems to maintain the unchanging consultation rates of general practice. There is a choice for GPs who can search through bewildering combinations of symptoms for the new epidemic illness, cancer and arterial disease, or for the universal problems of work, personal relationships and emotional development that lie behind so many physical complains. Of course most GPs look for both types of disorders as best they can, but the choice made by the academic vanguard reveals much about medical professionalism. They choose to concentrate on the search for psychological problems.

A school of psychological study developed in general practice, initated by a psychoanalyst called Michael Balint. and a group of GPs interested in the psychological aspects of medicine. This research stimulated more study and training, and came to dominate 'progressive' general practice and GP education. At its best it has given new, useful insights into the complex relationships between physical ailments and pscyhological and social problems, and has taught doctors new techniques for understanding and helping their patients. At its worst it has provided the vocabulary, and a superficial theory, to make old prejudices and ignorant assumptions appear respectably scientific. Psychological explanations for the problems that people bring to GPs are easier to make, and harder to test, than more orthodox physical explanations. In one sense, the Balint School and all that has flowed from it looks like an old tyrant in a new disguise – the judgements of the privileged, comfortable and efficient on the behaviour of the poor and distressed. Whatever the benefits and losses of this approach to medical care, it has replaced the more mechanical approach to disease processes. In doing so, it has conformed to the rules of medical professionalism. The focus of the new approach is on the individual patient and his/her problem, whilst the active agent is the watchful, thoughtful doctor.

Tradesman, customer and commodity are woven into the title of Michael Balint's most famous book, *The Doctor, His Patient and the Illness*. At the same time, other medical commodities have been diverted to other marketplaces, the supermarkets of the hospital network. Here, heart disease, cancers, high blood pressure, diabetes, epilepsy, arthritis and all the commonplace disorders are concentrated before specialist craftsmen trained to deal with them. In the hospitals diseases are ranked in order of value, like any other commodity. Everyday, often preventable but barely treatable diseases like chronic bronchitis generate little enthusiasm. Frail, elderly people with multiple, usually insoluble, problems, become the 'grot' and 'crumble' that 'block' the beds in acute surgical and medical wards that are needed for the better kinds of disease. Younger people with uncommon complaints are the best subject for the battery of investigative tests, skilled examinations and taxing, even heroic, surgery that may do them no good at all in the end, but which is a measure of their value to medicine. Hospitals are museums of pathology.

They were created both as sanctuaries for the ill and educational institutes for the rich. Scholarly gentlemen learned from the diseases of the poor, and applied their knowledge to their fee-paying clientele. It was the diseases rather than the poor that mattered, in 19th century hospitals. And in the 1980s medical students are still told to 'look at the liver in bed 7' or 'listen to the heart in bed 4'.

Our hospitals are not resources for their communities, even when they try to be. If they were, someone somewhere would have had to measure the needs of these communities, and then to direct the hospitals' activity towards meeting those needs. Vasectomies may be more necessary than varicose vein operations, and much more successful than cardiac surgery, but cardiac surgery will absorb the funds and vasectomy waiting lists will grow because needs are judged primarily from one standpoint – a medical one. People with diabetes will parade through hospital diabetic clinics for brief encounters with unfamiliar staff even though doing so may waste their time, make no difference to their diabetes or their general health, and use NHS resources fruitlessly. The doctor in the diabetic clinic may well know less about the patient's diabetes, and general health, between visits, than the patient does. S/he will know nothing about those queuing at bus-stops, pressing typewriter keys or propping up bars whose diabetes remains undiagnosed because they have not presented their symptoms to any health worker. Yet s/he and his or her colleagues will be the diabetic service for their community. Probably half of those with diabetes in Britain are unknown to the health service, and half of these known probably get minimal medical attention for a life-long, serious disease that threatens them with disability and premature death.

Those known and offered appropriate medical care may be lucky to get the full range of 'patient-centred' medicine. Their diseases will be monitored, their dietary options explained and their risk of complications reduced. Lasers may be used on their eyes when their sight is threatened, and a close watch kept for signs of arterial disease, heart strain or kidney failure. Even their backache or cystitis may be investigated, for underlying sexual problems, family conflicts or emotional disturbances. They will be the lucky recipients of the best medical science, and are more likely to be well-educated, moderately affluent and white, than poorly educated, on low incomes, or black. Their good fortune, if that is what it is, comes from their place in a commodity relationship and not from any accidental coincidence of problem and solution, nor any planned pursuit of preventable disease.

The Desirable and the Attainable

Medical care need not be organised like this. There is no good technical reason why the NHS cannot identity and try to help all or almost all of those with diabetes, heart diseases, arthritis, epilepsy, or any other serious disability or life-threatening disease. We know that health professionals can identify those at risk of a range of diseases, and intervene to prevent at least some people from crossing the threshold between risk and reality.

Cancer of the cervix kills 2,400 women a year in Britain. It is a preventable disease, and the overall UK death rate from it is falling. Yet the death rate amongst young women (aged between 25 and 34 years) is rising, and the number of young women in the population is also growing as the post-war boom generations grow up. Cervical cancer more commonly affects working class women, particularly if they have had several children. These women are exactly the group who do not, and probably cannot easily, make use of services for cervical cancer screening. If they did, their rate of premature death from cervical cancer would fall, for early detection allows early, and highly effective, treatment with laser techniques or surgery. Figure 14 shows the rising death rates from cervical cancer in young women in

Figure 14
Deaths From Cancer of the Cervix in Young Women Aged Between 25 and 34

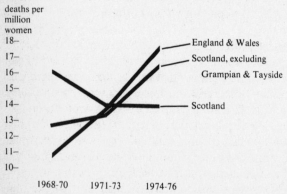

Source: Derived from Kate Gardner, 'Screening for Cervical Cancer', *Medicine in Society*, Vol. 8, No. 1.

Figure 15
Death Rates From Cancer of the Cervix in British Columbia, 1958-1974

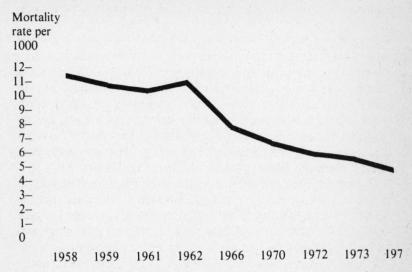

Source: Derived from Kate Gardner, 'Screening for Cervical Cancer',
Medicine in Society, Vol. 8, No. 1.

England and Wales, and the static death rate in Scotland. The
difference is caused by the impact of a well-organised screening
programme in the Grampian and Tayside area. When the
Grampian and Tayside death rates are subtracted from the rate
for all Scotland, the Scottish rate rises with the English.

Figure 15 shows the impact that long-term screening for
cancer of the cervic seems to have had in the Canadian Province
of British Columbia, compared with the UK.

Screening for cervical cancer is done by GPs, who are paid
for doing five-yearly screening tests done on women over 35, or
on those with 3 or more children, and also at antenatal,
postnatal and gynaecology clinics. That ought to allow those
most at risk to be reached, yet it does not seem to, probably
because of the limited use of NHS services made by women at
highest risk. A service that reaches out to them is needed – a
service that does not wait for them to find the time, enthusiasm
and courage to come forward, but actively offers itself on terms
convenient and acceptable to those in need.

Heart disease is responsible for nearly half of all deaths in
men before retirement age. It is not a disease of affluence, for it

affects the unskilled and semi-skilled worker more frequently than the professional or managerial workers, particularly amongst the younger age groups. Death rates from heart disease are 50% higher in Western Scotland, Northern Ireland and the South Wales mining valleys than they are in East Anglia and the affluent Home Counties, because of this class gap. Nor is it inevitable, for we know at least some of the factors that put individuals at risk from heart disease, and can intervene to minimise their impact. Control of high blood pressure, and the prevention of excessive and permanent rises in blood pressure would make a difference to the risk of heart disease. So would a reduction in cigarette smoking, and dietary changes that would reduce the levels of particular fats in the circulation.

Success has eluded the medical profession in its attempts to produce such changes, and failure is taken as evidence that the exercise is pointless. Yet the attempts have been poorly organised, inadequately funded and badly executed, and therefore doomed to failure. When people refuse to persist with life-long treatment of a risk like high blood pressure, in which there are no symptoms other than those produced as side-effects by meditation, it is easier to blame them for 'poor compliance' – for being ignorant and disobedient – than to blame their doctors for being poor communicators, advisors and persuaders. If we continue to smoke cigarettes, despite all warnings, we are wilfully risking our health, and not responding to the multiple forces that prompt us to smoke. Here professionalism fuses with fantasy. The 'bad patient' is the person who rejects commodities offered by the tradesman. He or she should go to another shop, and not waste the doctor's time.

Failure is no obstacle to medical intervention when the market benefits. Heart transplantation is pursued as a technique because of its possibilities, despite its cost in lives and cash. More modest heart surgery may work for some with heart disease, but it will not help most of those affected – yet cardiac surgeons prosper and thrive, whilst preventive approaches stumble at the first obstacles. The industries that make electrocardiograms, cardiac-shock machines, ventilators, transfusion and cooling equipment, and X-ray cameras have no interest in reducing blood fat levels by dietary changes. The cardiac surgeons developing their private practice in a growing market will not abandon their immense technical skills to combat smoking. And neither the doctor nor his or her patient can resist the illness, once it has appeared as a commodity within their market relationship. It is not heart disease that is inevitable, but its belated treatment by largely ineffective methods.

Drugs – A Financial Addiction

Prominent amongst medicine's ineffective methods is the use of drugs. The modern pharmaceutical industry explains its importance in terms of the demand it meets, the jobs it creates, the profits it makes and recirculates, the exports it sells, and last of all, the necessities it produces. The stream of 'new' drugs born as their predecessors' patents expire, of multiple variations on basic formulae, and of dazzling choices between virtually identical brands, makes the pharmaceutical industry more economically than socially useful. Yet the drugs industry completes the market relationship between doctor and patient, playing the role of wholesaler to the tradesman and his customer, and seeking to influence both in their decisions.

The prime target for the pharmaceutical industry is the doctor, and other health professionals (pharmacists, district nurses, health visitors) who can influence doctors. The doctor-drug company relationship is a cosy one, and much less uncomfortable than the doctor-patient relationship. One estimate put the cost of drug promotion for each GP as equal to the cost of paying a pharmacologist to retrain the doctor in the use of drugs for one month each year. A study in 1974-75 showed that GPs were then exposed to 1,300 adverts for 250 different preparations, each month. In 1977 the drug companies spent £71 million on sales promotion, the bulk of it aimed at GPs. At 1979 prices, the average doctor can expect to have £30,000 spent on his or her 'postgraduate education' by the drugs industry – about twice the cost of his or her original education. Britain's 150 medical journals derive 40-60% of their income from drug company advertising, and forty or so 'free papers', with frequency varying from weekly to monthly, are entirely financed by drug advertising. The pharmaceutical industry funds scientific and educational meetings, providing free food and drink and contributing to advertising costs and speakers expenses, in return for promotional displays and the showing of advertising films.

The relationship works. In 1979 doctors wrote 370 million

prescriptions for medicines costing £750 million, and the profits on the sales totalled £125 million. In 1980 the profit rate on drug sales to the NHS was 21%, with some companies showing nearer 30%. By comaprison the pre-tax return for the chemical industry as a whole was 18.2%, and for all manufacturing industry it was 17.6%. Only advertising and oil were more profitable than drug production, and that was during a bad phase for the industry. Between 1968 and 1972 the UK pharmaceutical industry grew at an annual rate of 10% – at least 3 times the growth rate of all manufacturing industry. The high level of profit derives from its privileged position in relation to its main buyer, the NHS. Whilst there is competition between companies, all are agreed on the two basic principles of drug marketing: the intensive promotion of expensive brand-name drugs; and the concentration of the promotion on drugs not yet widely used, or on medications of dubious value.

The *Daily Telegraph* ran an interesting story about drug industry profiteering in its issue of 27 November 1979.

> Millions of pounds annually are added needlessly to the NHS drugs bill by mass prescribing of expensive brand-named tablets which are available more cheaply under other names.
>
> Thirteen brand leaders among the most widely prescribed drugs all also available in cheaper form, added at least £25 million unnecessarily to the 1978 drug bill of £723 million.
>
> Of these 13 brands, five costs twice as much as their unbranded equivalents, three cost 4, 6 and 10 times more respectively than their equivalents, while the remaining five were between 78-40% more.

The debate about the costs of brand-name versus chemical-name (generic) medicines prompted a government enquiry, initiated by Tory Social Services Secretary, Patrick Jenkin, and chaired by the DHSS's Chief Medical Advisor, Dr Peter Greenfield. The Greenfield Committee reported to Ministers in February 1982, but its conclusions were not formally made public that year. Leaks from the DHSS suggested that the report recommended generic substitution. This would allow chemists to substitute cheaper, generic, preparations for expensive brand-name products unless specifically instructed not to by the prescribing doctor. Junior Health Minister, Geoffrey Finsbery, told Tory MP, Janet Fookes, in December 1982 that 'overall savings to the NHS would be very small indeed'. The *Guardian* reported on 29 December 1982 that independent research suggested a saving of 10% on the 1982 drug bill of £1,700 million if generic substitution was extended from the hospitals (where it already operated) to general practice. The £170 million saved would have been enough to provide intensive care for every premature baby needing it *and* enough kidney dialysis units to save the lives of 7,000 people with kidney failure. The BMA took part in the Greenfield enquiry, and favours generic substitution provided that it is *not* compulsory. The professional argued for an escape clause, allowing doctors to *insist* on brand-name products when they felt it would benefit their patient, and got what they wanted. Such an escape clause would be no great problem for the drugs industry, which would intensify its efforts to demonstrate the unique and essential properties of each branded pill and capsule.

The Hard Sell

That intensified promotional campaign would be only an extension of current practice. Drugs well-established on the market need little advertising, and neither do standard medicines of proven value. Neither the common tranquillisers, prescribed in millions, nor drugs used for the treatment of diabetes get much advertising space unless rivals appear or patents lapse. The lavish promotion is reserved for drugs with huge market potential but of dubious clincial merit – antacids for indigestion, cough and cold mixtures, another new answer for arthritis, yet another remedy for depression. These drugs have 14-15% of their total cost spent on their promotion, compared with 1.9% for the standard treatment for diabetes.

Drug promotion aims to encourage chemical solutions for the problems presented to doctors, irrespective of the genuine medical content of these problems. One Swiss company, Sandoz, marketed a new tranquilliser recently, saying it was for: 'The anxiety which comes from not fitting in – the newcomer in town who can't make friends – the woman who can't get along with her daughter-in-law – the executive who can't accept retirement'. The drug firm Roche responded to the growing mass obsession about sleeplessness by coining the expression 'The Sleep Cripple', telling general practitioners that 'proper sleep' was necessary to prevent a nervous breakdown. The pharmaceutical industry rapidly exploited and encouraged unrealistic fears about sleeplessness, and has profited from the sale of sleeping tablets. These drugs rapidly lose their chemical sleep-inducing effect but they induce psychological dependence, so that people cannot sleep without them, and they provoke distressing side-effects – particularly sleep disturbance – when stopped. Through the cultivation of fear and the promotion of an ineffective solution to an artificial problem, the pharmaceutical industry recruits lifelong clients. Some of these clients' lives are also terminated with the industry's products; Age Concern reports that two-thirds of accidental deaths among those over 65 are due to taking sleeping tablets.

Should the medical profession, busy defending its autonomy against all except the drugs industry, prove an unreliable market-organiser for new medicines, the mass media can be used. The industry's technique is to present its new drugs to the press, particularly the headline-hungry popular dailies that lap-up 'miracle drug' stories, to encourage premature and exaggerated publicity. Instead of simply projecting the new drug's image through the medical press, direct-mail advertising and individual lobbying of doctors by company representatives, the public is enrolled to act as free advocates of the latest innovation. The industry can claim that it is acting in the public interest by disseminating educative information, and deplore the distortions and exaggerations introduced by tabloids engaged in cut-throat circulation wars. In the last resort, the doctors can be condemned for their weakness in prescribing what their patients want, whilst the promoting company retains its self-proclaimed worth as an honest public servant.

In fact the unreliability of doctors as middlemen for the industry is growing, and prompting the public marketing techniques. A letter in the *British Medical Journal* of 3 November 1979 complained bitterly about the way Sandoz had launched their new anti-asthma drug, Ketotifen.

> ... A national press release, organised by inviting journalists to a briefing outside the UK, has stimulated many patients to ask their doctors to prescribe this drug for them ... doctors are being persuaded to prescribe by adverts which rely on manifestly inadequate evidence and in which the dangers of the treatment appear in very small print. Furthermore, GPs are being offered £15

for each patient for whom a history card and three-month follow-up form are completed.

The growing refusal by GPs to deal with drug company representatives is a small, but irritating act of resistance that annoys the industry. So too are schemes for reviewing prescribing habits so that drugs can be used more rationally, and at less expense to the NHS. The cooperation of the BMA with the Greenfield enquiry, and its qualified support of genetic substitution, are worrying signs for the drugs industry. They do not yet threaten profits, but they demonstrate that the medical profession is pulled two ways. Its own individualist philosophy, and its market origins, tie it to its suppliers and make it an effective middleman. Its incorporation into a collective system of health care, however imperfect, with a whole population perspective, however poorly expressed, makes it adopt at least some public interests as its own. Medicine cannot afford to be stigmatised as junior partner to a profit-hungry and relatively unscrupulous industry. Nor can the profession ignore government pressure for economy measures within health care, for the doctors' incomes themselves come from the public purse. The medical profession is not in danger of defecting into the socialist camp, and the drug companies need not panic. Nevertheless, alarming possibilities exist for separating the middlemen and their suppliers, and the drugs industry will work hard during the eighties to strengthen its influence over medicine, aided enthusiastically by the profession's conservatives.

The RCN

The options inherent within medicine exist in the other health professions. In some respects they can appear more clearly because these professions are subordinate to medicine in both their work-organisation and their access to power, and can rebel against their subordination. On the other hand the overwhelmingly female composition of their membership has militated against substantial change, except when directed by a conventional and thoroughly middle-class leading echelon. Nursing is the obvious example. The Royal College of Nursing has captured the bulk of the skilled nursing workforce, accounting for 180,000 NHS nurses (including the majority of nursing students), and has doubled its membership since 1977, despite its deliberate policy of excluding nursing assistants and nursing auxiliaries. It has been able to express a truly professional concern with developing skills appropriate to market relationships, by meeting the demand for specialist education that grew out of the 'nursing process' boom of the sixties and seventies. Its exclusion of unskilled nursing labour, designed to separate the professional skills from the menial tasks in nursing, permitted trade union recruitment amongst nurses, but (until very recently) confined that trade unionism to the traditional industrial role of defending workers' interests.

The RCN, like the BMA, has used its professionalism as a base from which it can try and control the theory and practice of 'public service'. Its hostility to industrial action may have given it an excuse for staying outside the TUC, but it has become an independent certified trade union with a large labour relations department supporting a network of full-time officers covering every region. One of the reasons for the RCN's remarkable growth in the late seventies is its effective combination of professional attitudes and trade union organisation. Trade unions like COHSE and NUPE, on the other hand, have no such professional advantages. Their natural bases are either amongst nursing auxiliaries and assistants (NUPE) or in the mental illness and mental handicap hospitals where nursing care differs substantially from that in DGHs, and where there is a significant male workforce (COHSE). TUC-affiliated unions will have to evolve strategies towards professionalism if they are to break out from their traditional areas of support and undermine the RCN's influence. And to do that they may have to overcome serious internal conflicts, like the understandable resistance of COHSE members to the run-down of large mental illness hospitals or to the reform of nursing education for the care of mentally handicapped.

The game is going the professionals' way, even though the beginning of the 1982 pay campaign suggested that the unions were the dominant force. That does not necessarily mean that a collectivist approach cannot influence the health professions in the eighties. There are strains within orthodox professionalism that may neutralise the impact of Conservatism on health care, if exploited by the labour movement. The problem is, is the labour movement up to it?

CHAPTER 8
Class, Consumerism and Resources

We are approaching another turning point in the politics of health. Those of us who defend social provision against the market need a new philosophy to guide a new political practice and a new economic approach to health services, if our arguments are to survive. We will have to learn from our own history, not because it has the answers, but because it teaches the questions.

Britain is now poor in socialist philosophy. Our traditions are dominated by idealism, by preoccupations with causes and their effects, by an intense belief in willpower, and by a passion for the correct policy for each neat problem. Ideas of central planning, of careful analysis, and of powerful social policy have created an enormous state that attempts to shape and govern the evolving market economy. The Fabian notion of a society engineered by sound decisions and effective instruments, according to a thoughtful plan drawn up by the educated on behalf of the ignorant, has been of enormous benefit to us. It has been an antidote to those who turn commodity-exchange into a religion, measuring the value of everything and exploiting every weakness methodically, cruelly and thoroughly. It created the National Health Service, the Welfare State and the consumer society. And now it is beginning to fail, as its own foundation, the power and affluence of Britain in the world, declines.

The idealist, liberal view of health is simple. Health is a state that can be achieved, if you do the right things. Ill health comes from low incomes, poor housing and inadequate education. Malnutrition, overwork, reduced resistance and ignorance mediate between these casual factors and their effects – tuberculosis, heart disease, syphilis, depression, polio, madness, handicap and premature death. The 'right things' are the policies and actions that eradicate the causes and subsequently their mediators, whilst organising the efficient disposal of their effects.

Legislation is the key weapon, aimed at universal education, welfare benefits, free health care, subsidised food, safety at work, continued economic expansion and (nearly) full employment. Strategies and strategists are needed to create the legislation, and mechanisms (with mechanics) are needed to carry out the programmes. Politics is the range of strategies, the choice of mechanisms. The state becomes a huge machine, ordering and organising its society according to blueprint. For Beveridge and his colleagues, the new state and its welfare policies would eradicate disease. The health service would devour the backlog of unmet need, and the burden of illness would decrease. The NHS would undermine its own reason for existence, and perhaps even wither away.

None of these hopes materialised, but their instruments of delivery have. We have a Welfare State, yet widespread poverty persists. We have public education, and the class gap in knowledge stays wide. The National Health Service grows yearly, yet new diseases replace the old ones, and builders are still less healthy than architects. Behind it all, the economy declines. The consequences for idealism, and for the liberal philosophy of health, are a classic example of social psychology. When any strongly-held belief is exposed as false, some of its adherents abandon it, and perhaps all other beliefs too, in favour of scepticism and cynicism. Others, however, redouble their conviction. Both have occurred in health care, with the former response dominant.

As it became obvious that the Beveridge idea of decreasing illness was unrealistic, the right regained the initiative. Their answer to the problem was a market slogan – 'infinite demand, finite resources'. Illness would not disappear, to socialist order, because it was the population's subjective desire for medical care that created 'illness', and not the bacteria, neuroses, hormones and cancer cells described by science. Within the population was an urge to sit in surgeries, talk to doctors, have X-rays and blood tests, and undergo operations, that was insatiable. Existentialist philosophy rescued market economics to explain how consumers of health services used modern medical magic to minimise the pain of human existence. Since mortality was inescapable, state-run health services had to resist consumer demands, except where necessary provision was required. What constituted 'necessity' could be determined by suitable combinations of professional judgement, consumer demand and suppliers' capacities. This line of argument was not restricted to the Conservative Party, and was adopted by Liberal and Labour politicians too. Nor does it necessarily work to the medical profession's advantage.

Women deliver their babies into baths of lukewarm water, whilst squatting through labour pains and drinking herbal remedies, because they prefer to, not because it is really safer, wiser or more natural than any other form of birth. They may well have paid private midwives, and perhaps private doctors too, to legitimise this experiment. Their justification will come from first or second-hand experience of powerlessness and humiliation at the hands of NHS obstetricians and midwives, ideas of natural body rhythms, and perhaps assorted mystical beliefs. They may leave today's 'pompous trades and proud mechanics', the technological-minded obstetricians, speechless with rage, but they also conform to the rules of consumerism in health care, and demonstrate the extent of demand and its power to influence supplies. 'Natural' chidlbirth is one extreme example of consumerism.

The educated middle class, as a whole, gets better service from the NHS because of its aptitude for such consumerism. The USA has more stringent legislation controlling new industrial chemicals, new foodstuff ingredients and new medicines than the UK because US consumers (including the US trade unions) are better organised and pack more punch in the marketplace. Those are positive advantages that puzzle those who think that a relatively unrestricted market economy cannot tolerate complex and effective social provision. These advantages stem, however, from a consumer ethic, and are double-edged. When social provision becomes 'too expensive', and of less weight in the market relationship, it can be replaced by the ethics of individual responsibility. Then health depends on *individuals* doing the right things whether that is eating bran, jogging, or having babies in the bath. 'Look after yourself' is the philosophy of the consumer, and can be applied collectively or individually, according to the state of the market. (It was also the theme of a recent Health Education Council campaign, and is the unwritten slogan of the private sector in health care).

Health as Consumerism

The over-riding aim of Conservatism is to turn us all into consumers of health services, regardless of the inconsistencies in their approach. Private medicine is the obvious example, but every Health Authority incorporates consumerism into its routine planning and activity. The idea of cash-limits to budgets fosters conflicts between departments and disciplines for available money. Charity walks, swims and parachute jumps raise money for the favoured, prestigious facility – body scanners, kidney dialysis machines, special care incubators – rather than for extra nurses, midwives, geriatric beds or community homes that may be more useful, but that are also less appealing. Trade unionists seeking pay increases are told that their extra pay must come out of someone else's budget, and that the ill *must* suffer if the health workers are to keep head above water.

In some senses we appear to gain from this consumerism. The women's movement has had an enormous impact on NHS activity, retaining abortion services when pressure has increased against them, and in places like Merseyside and Manchester developing new services (daycare abortion units and well woman clinics) against strong opposition. Yet its impact has come, in part at least, through its operation as the biggest consumer group in the country, as well as through the alliance built between women's organisations and the trade union movement. That is not, in itself, a bad thing. On the contrary, the separate identity of the women's movement, and the separate expression of women's interests, are essential for the development of democracy.

The problems begin when consumer interests are answered, in true market style, according to their market power. For the NHS administration, an organised and energetic force of vocal, educated young women rightly seeking proper family planning facilities has one weight. Professional and commercial voices that speak in favour of new technology have a second weight. The mass of retired people who accept, often unnecessarily, deterioration in their health, are a third. How can planners, Finance Officers, or Health Authority members decide priorities? In practice, they can only compare the weights, measuring the strengths of contesting interests. They could, and in some case they do, confront the applicants for resources with a predetermined plan of allocation based on national needs. But they rarely, if ever, enrol *all* the interest groups in deciding the plan, or carrying it out. If they did, the consumerism of this or that interest group would wither as each accepts a social responsibility. Juggling NHS priorities, and balance sheets, is the consequence of a conservative consumerism in health care, and has dominated planning.

The RAWP formula, whatever its faults, was an effort at planning. Between 1976 and 1979, only 5 of the 14 RHAs applied the RAWP methods, and even then were cautious in establishing targets for specific services. Four Regions were not able to analyse their populations according to average death rates, and five had not worked out their hospital requirements. Fabianism, projecting its social plan drawn up by experts, appears in the careful forward thinking of Oxford Region – the pre-eminent Region in England and Wales for its planned approach to health services, and the first Region to realise that a comprehensive service and Conservataive government cash-limits were incompatible.

If the idealism fails and consumerism triumphs, long live idealism. Since decision-making in the NHS has fallen into the hands of the opposition, the best thing an idealist can do is abandon it as lost ground. A new strategy can then emerge, discounting the lost territories. Health services, we relearn, do not usually make much difference to the duration of our lives. Social conditions are the deciding factors, and our new, wider strategy is aimed at changing them. If the average building worker is to have the same life expectancy, and the same pattern of health, as the architect, he must also have the same standards of housing, income, and education, the same amount and kind of work, a similar diet, and similar habits. The unemployed young single mother with one or two toddlers, living ten floors up in a high-rise block, will need the same income, education, quality of housing, density of social relations and quantity of child-care support as her journalist sister living in a gentrified Victorian terraced house (with garden) only a few hundred yards away, if she is to live as long and as well. Health services are part of the fine detail in the pictures, curing occasionaly, consoling often and caring always. They are, in fact, luxuries compared with sewers, wholesome food, spacious homes and good education.

'Capitalism Makes you Ill'. Does it?

The wider strategy is sound, but old. It is less sound than it was in the 18th and 19th centuries, but it retains much force and appeal. Those casting around for strategic inspiration often gain strength from starker situations that emulate a clear-cut past. Socialist Mozambique, China and Cuba are the inspirations for 'new' philosophies of health care, whilst East Germany, Finland, Czechoslovakia, Sweden or the USSR are merged with the grey, unhelpful industrialised world. Doctors interested in disease enthuse over the gross pathology seen in the Third World. Radicals enthuse at the measures to eradicate gross pathology: the barefoot doctor (cheap medical care for an expendable peasantry), the mass campaigns against snails, or mosquitoes, or for more hygienic sewage disposal. Each group pursues its own interests, expressed through other nations' experiences in a way that only a long colonial tradition could create. Back home, where the situation is much more complex, idealism has two options. The first is utopian, blaming capitalism for both creating and profiting from ill health. The second is reductionist, constricting the problems to fit a narrow solution.

The idea that capitalism makes you ill depends on three arguments. The first is that the market economy creates inequalities in social conditions, which in turn create inequalities in health. The second is that the profit motive can, and does, overrule health considerations. The third is that medical care is closely related to the market economy, or even part of it, and is of less real value than its practitioners claim – it is a professional conspiracy against the public. All three arguments are true, as far as they go, and they seem to support the overall theme of capitalism as a cause of ill health. Unfortunately, they are incomplete, and their consequences are not always what their authors hope. First of all, the arguments omit any active role for people. The acceptance of a social order, with its inequalities and hierarchies, by the subordinate classes is often left out of socialist thinking. It is an unpleasant thought that, say, an industrial working class could opt for a consumer society rather than a socialist economy, and marxists may be forgiven for their attachment to conspiracy theories. Nevertheless, the values of social groups and classes determine their political responses, and those values are interpretations of collective experience. 'So what?' is a reasonable answer to the assertion that 'capitalism makes you ill', since an older generation will testify that it once made you much worse! The fact that the building worker and the architect experience different patterns of health illness may be outweighed by their acceptance of their unequal status, and of the improvements each has to show, compared with his parents. Whilst progress seems possible with the old methods, why abandon them, particularly when the alternatives seem unappetising? If progress seems blocked, however, then individual and collective attitudes may change, and new responses occur. The exclusion of the people from an active role in maintaining the social structure occurs because idealist philosophy does not begin where people are, but where they should be.

If capitalism makes you ill, then socialism will presumably make you less ill, or not ill at all. From the three arguments, socialism is a social order without inequalities in social conditions, without the profit motive, and with a much reduced need for medical care. The underlying assumption here is of abundance – abundance that negates the need for surplus value, and abundance that makes inequality in the distribution of resources unnecessary. Whilst the world's resources may more than meet the world's needs, if used for that purpose, we have no real prospect of achieving that abundance in the foreseeable future. The country with the greatest wealth, the USA, is the least socialist, whilst the socialist countries are either amongst the poorest, or are recent victims of devastating wars, or both.

What use to us is an idea that presupposes abundance, when we will have to accept and work within scarcity, inequality and the need for surplus value? In practice, it has many uses. It may repeat the Beveridge dream that once the social policies are implemented, the problem will be solved. Eliminate capitalism, and illness will diminish and the medical profession shrink. It may demonstrate that, since abundance is unobtainable, inequality and the pursuit of profit should be accepted uncritically. It can be turned round, so that if you are ill, you must be suffering from capitalism. Then illness is a marker for capitalism, and all those countries claiming to be socialist can be exposed for what they really are – state capitalism. At best, the rhetoric can be dropped in favour of more modest conclusions. Social conditions influence health, and Tory governments make us ill because they foster unemployment, tolerate hazardous work conditions and create social stress. A socialist government would have transport, housing, education and industrial policies that would do more to favour health. So it should, but the argument has turned full circle, and we are back where we began, considering the people's judgement on options open to them. The options now are different from those of 1911 and 1948, for no-one is promising to open up access to the services previously denied to people. Instead we have a choice, between our experience of (and ignorance about) our present circumstances and the promise of improved health through changes in ways of living. Are people wrong to reject abstract future advantages in favour of current realities?

Chemical Risk

If the wider strategy appear unimpressive to the public, perhaps it is time to narrow it down? If socialism isn't the cure for illness, maybe macrobiotic foods or homoeopathy are more likely to promote health? Narrower still, perhaps we can control the modern epidemic of cancer by eradicating the dangerous cancer-inducing chemicals used so widely in industry. This is an alternative approach. It identifies a general and alarming problem, locates an identifiable cause for it, and offers a solution through existing mechanisms. People fear cancer, and see it as a single disease with many disguises. More and more individuals seem to suffer with it and die from it, and it has come to symbolise pain, suffering and sadness. Some chemicals are known to cause cancer, and more are suspects.

Industry, in the market economy, has a poor record when it comes to dangerous chemicals, and uses its workers (and consumers) for experiments in chemical safety. From the point of view of the market, new and profitable chemicals are safe until proved otherwise through the disability of death of those handling or using them. The onus of proof can often be left to the victims, as well, and where there is doubt, the chemical can be exonerated and the victim blamed. From the standpoint of the industrial worker, or the user of the product, the reverse is true. New chemicals are dangerous until proved otherwise, simply because so many have been in the past. The onus of proof of safety lies with those who gain from introducing the new chemical, and whilst there is any doubt about hazards, safety is not proven. The scene is set for a full-scale clash of interests, between those putting profit first, and those putting health first.

The Trade union movement rightly takes the cautious attitude, defending not only its own members' interests, but also trying to defend those consuming industrial goods, living in industrial areas, or exposed to avoidable hazards. The farmworkers' campaign against the pesticide 245-T is the well-publicised tip of the iceberg of trade union activity aimed at increasing health and safety in and around industry. The temptation for the trade union movement is to extend the general argument, and present the control of industrial chemical hazards as *the* solution to the apparent epidemic of cancer. For the left, this view can be a political face-saver. It identifies the cause and solution to a major, perhaps the major, health hazard as being outside the territory of health care. It also gives the trade union movement a powerful role in putting the situation right, provides

Figure 16
Death Rates From Cancers – Annual Death Rates From Common Cancers Amongst Men and Women Aged Between 45 and 64

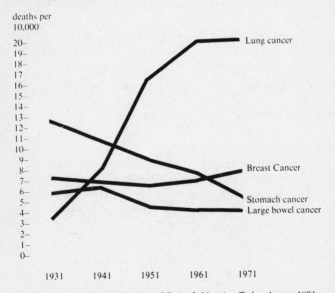

Source: Dave Forman. 'The Politics of Cancer'. *Marxism Today*. August 1981.

a new reason for winning the conflict between capital and labour and may even teach that the industrial workforce remains a political vanguard, the cutting-edge of change. Unfortunately, the argument is over-extended. Cancers are widespread causes of illness and death, partly because of a dramatic increase in lung cancer and partly because other illness that once killed people before they could develop any form of cancer, has declined. Figure 16 shows death rates from several cancers, over a forty year period.

Smoking, East and West

There are good reasons for blaming environmental factors, including industrial hazards and pollution for the development of cancers. There is a good case for controlling the use of potentially-hazardous chemicals to *try* and reduce the overall incidence of cancer, and there is no doubt that the onus of proving safety must be on those who profit from industrial production, whether they be a private company or a nationalised industry. None of these arguments add up to the view that the answer to cancer lies with trade union control of industrialised processes. On the contrary, consumption of hazardous products is a much more serious cause of disease, and the leading factor in promoting cancer-development is certainly cigarette smoking.

Tobacco-processing is a highly profitable industry, of value to its owners, to a government needing tax revenues, to its industrial workforce (particularly in a recession), and to the consuming public (48% of adult men and 38% of adult women, in 1976). Yet the social value of reducing tobacco consumption would be enormous. Industry itself pays for cigarette smoking through lost production due to sickness absence, impaired productivity due to poor health, and material damage from accidents and fires attributable to smoking. The Royal College of Physicians estimates that smoking results in the loss of 50 million working days a year – four times the number lost through industrial action. In 1979 nearly 20% of all fires in industrial premises were due to smoking materials, whilst a survey of industrial accidents demonstrated a higher accidental rate amongst smokers than amongst non-smokers. Each year over 50,000 people die before retirement age, as a direct result of smoking tobacco. The three major diseases caused by cigarette smoking are lung cancer, chronic bronchitis and heart disease. Cigarette smoking is the cause in 90% of lung cancer deaths, whilst 95% of chronic bronchitis sufferers are smokers. One quarter of premature deaths from heart disease are caused by smoking. Figure 17 shows the numbers of deaths from cigarette-related diseases, in 1978.

Figure 17
Cigarette-Related Deaths

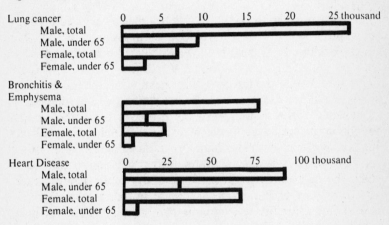

Source: Tom Hurst, 'Smoking and Health', *Medicine in Society*, Vol. 8, No. 4.

Smoking is a class-related habit, and smoking-related diseases are more frequent within working class populations. The number of smokers is declining, but faster amongst professionals than amongst manual workers. In 1980, only 25% of male, and slightly fewer female, professionals smoked, whilst 57% of male and 41% of female unskilled manual workers were smokers. The costs to the NHS of treating smoking-related diseases is difficult to measure, but the Labour Secretary of State, David Ennals, estimated that in 1977 the health service spent £2 million a week on such treatments. The costs to the Exchequer in payment of invalidity pensions, widows benefits and Social Security benefits to dependents, are unknown.

In tobacco-related diseases we have an excellent example of conventional wisdom applied to people's health, with disastrous consequences. Blaming smokers for smoking is an everyday hypocrisy perpetrated by governments which benefit from taxation on the tobacco industry's profits, and whose predecessors helped create a market by endorsing the healthy, relaxing qualities of smoking. The tobacco industry has no real interest in reducing its profits. The industry's workforce (and the trade union movement generally) do not make campaigns against smoking a priority issue, and the consuming public has shown no enthusiasm for allegedly safe products (like New Smoking Material – NSM). Health education works, but mostly amongst those already highly educated. Sometimes it has a contrary effect, appearing as yet another middle-class imposition on working-class habits. A 40% reduction in cigarette consumption (less than that already achieved amongst male professional workers) would result in a saving of 30 million lost working days, and bout 8,500 lives each year. Such a health-conserving measure seems worthwhile, but is it currently too expensive for the UK market to bear.

Nor can we assume that abolition of private ownership in tobacco production will solve the problem. the USSR has an advanced health education programme directed against tobacco consumption that is better than any mounted in the West, except perhaps for Sweden's. Soviet tobacco production increased by 69% between 1960 and 1980, and the tenth five-year plan (1976-80) anticipated a 20% increase in output over the 1975 level. Consumption of cigarettes rose rapidly in the sixties to now match West European levels, is two thirds of US and UK consumption per head, and has required importation of West European processing machinery and Bulgaria tobacco. A major survey of smoking habits in six Soviet cities, published in 1981, found that 48% of men aged 40-59 years were smokers, and that smoking was related to educational level. Only 37% of those with higher education were smokers, compared with 60% of those with secondary education, and 65% of those with only primary-level education. The number of lung cancer deaths almost doubled from 1960 to 1975, rising from 24,500 to 57,000, with death rates highest in Republics with the highest tobacco consumption. Heart disease increased by an average of 7% a year during the sixties and early seventies – a rate of increase greater than previously recorded in any other country. Whilst this unprecedented rise in heart disease is not entirely related to tobacco consumption, heavy smoking increases the risk of heart disease by more than two-fold.

The USSR faces a chronic labour shortage, and has many reasons to pursue a health provision policy, but these appear to be offset by other economic and social considerations. The value of the tobacco crop rose by more than 100%, from 234 million roubles in 1960 to 542 million roubles in 1975. The money generated for government use from this increased value is unknown, but like alcohol production, tobacco contributes direct revenue. Cigarettes also contribute to consumer goods output, being a highly marketable commodity requiring relatively little investment in technology and industrial plant. Smoking cigarettes, like eating a high fat diet, has become part of the Soviet effort to catch up with the West. It is what the people want, and its in the government's interest to meet those wants.

The Soviet experience does noì mean that tobacco consumption is inevitable or unalterable, although the industry may pretend that it does. It does demonstrate that the simple approach of centralists, initiating change through government action, does not work with complex problems. The government is not above the problem, but part of it. It does not act independently of the needs of industry or the society, and it has to resolve contradictions between antagonistic public needs. In the field of health and health care, that applies to both capitalist and socialist governments. The Soviet experience is easy to understand in the context of its very rapid development from Third World status to superpower, but that still does not negate the principles involved. Only by denying that the USSR is socialist can we maintain the myth that socialism will solve our current problems, and then we have only hopes, dreams and the thoughts of assorted prophets, past and present.

If we look more carefully at the Soviet experience, we can see their real, natural advantages. A centrally-planned economy allows, in principle at least, for the substitution of one profitable but hazardous commodity with another equally profitable, but less hazardous, one. The transformation of wants, through extension of higher education throughout the society, is also easier when economic planning allots an appropriate priority to educational spending. Change remains dependent on political pressure. If a Soviet 'tobacco lobby' exists, it must operate through the political machinery to influence decision-making, and oppose a health-promotion lobby, or perhaps Treasury pressure for limiting health service spending. How the Soviet political machine *really* works may be unclear, but the message we get is clear enough. Central economic and social planning provides a mechanism for continuous social change, and political debate within it, between different interests and viewpoints, determined the direction and pace of change. Socialism is not then a solution, but an opportunity.

Obstacles to Change

The liberal philosophy abandons opportunities in health politics. By rejecting political pressure within health professionalism, the whole territory is conceded to the right. Confrontations can occur at the boundaries of the territory: managers are organised against doctors; some within the women's movement attack male professionalism over attitudes, services and omissions; ancillary workers clash with consultants over pay beds; trade unionists refuse to sit alongside professional organisation representatives in joint staff consultative committees and professional bodies try to exclude unions from wage negotiations. We pay a high price for shaping health politics this way.

Professionals, left to themselves, do what they are accustomed to do, and they try to do it well. Whether it works, or is for the best, is not the issue. It has evolved from within professionalism's body of knowledge and skills, and when no

Figure 18
Death Rates of Children Aged Under 15, From Diptheria

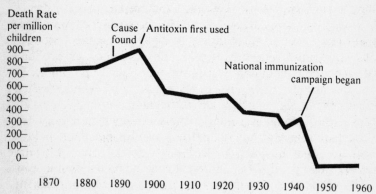

Source: T. McKeown, *The Role of Medicine*, 1979.

pressures are applied, professionals change their methods slowly. That may be a necessary antidote to a commercial enthusiasm for novelty, but it also delays useful innovation. Let's take an example cited by a good representative of the liberal tradition, Thomas McKeown, as evidence that good social conditions are more important than medical services in determining health – diptheria. Death rates from diptheria were rising, until diptheria antitoxin was developed and used in 1895, as Figure 18 shows.

Death rates fell after the introduction of antitoxin, and although McKeown doubts that this was due solely to treatment, he cannot deny its role. What he misses out from his analysis is the time-lapse between the discovery of effective immunisation and is wide-scale use. Immunisation to prevent a child catching diptheria was developed in 1913. Its general use was advocated by the Chief Medical Officer to the new Ministry of Health in 1922, but it was not until 1940 that mass immunisation began. For 18 years about 3,000 children died each year from a preventable disease. The medical response, between 1922 and 1940, was to refine its skills, diagnosing diptheria once caught, treating it with antitoxin, admitting affected chidlren to special wards in infectious diseases hospitals, and creating artificial openings in the throat when the disease threatened to asphyxiate its victim. At the same time, immunisation was defined as a medical task, beyond others' skills. Because professional expertise was unchallengeable, an opportunity to implement an important preventive measure was delayed. Had there been a more powerful pressure-group within medicine, advocating change, and acting in concert with broader political interests, perhaps that delay might have been shorter, and fewer lives lost unnecessarily?

Handicapped Babies, a Case in Point

More recently, emphasis on the social factors determining our health had benefited the Thatcher government, when it was under pressure to expand maternity services. In 1978 the Spastics Society launched a campaign to reduce the number of babies dying, or suffering handicap, at birth. This campaign prompted an investigation by a House of Common Select Committee, chaired by Renee Short, MP. The Short Report on perinatal and neonatal mortality was published in July 1980, and concluded that the application of modern medical knowledge and technical care to all pregnant women would prevent 3-5,000 deaths, and another 5,000 cases of handicap, each year. It made 152 recommendations that it costed at only £25 million, and estimated a saving of £152 million over 10 years through the prevention of handicap. Many of these recommendations were based on assumptions that the only way to reduce mortality was by centralising services and applying high-technology medicine to pregnancy and labour. The committee appeared to have been influenced by both obstetricians and the medical supply industry. One committee member, speaking at the Report's press conference, described the technology needed as 'fine British products' and spelled out the name of the major British manufacturer, Sonicaid, to the journalists present.

The government's reply in December 1980 rejected key proposals in the Report, on several counts. Firstly, the government rightly argued that the Select Committee had overestimated the impact medical care could have in preventing death or handicap. Without having detailed facts about the frequency of handicaps, and the number of handicapped babies whose disability could be attributed to birth-problems, the Select Committee assumed that measures taken to prevent death would also prevent handicap. There is little evidence to support this view, and indeed there is a reasonable argument for the opposition opinion – the more premature babies supported in intensive care units, the more handicapped infants there will be. The Select Committee went on to argue, without providing evidence, that the social disadvantages causing death at or around birth could be overcome by well-directed medical intervention. The government opted, in its reply, for the conclusions reached by the Baird Committee in its study of perinatal problems in Ireland.

Many of the factors which affect the outcome of pregnancy lie outside the traditional scope of the health services ... we believe that prevention of death and handicap begins in the socio-economic sphere ... greater prosperity, full employment and adequate housing would in themselves make a larger impact on the problem than would changes in the nature and organisation of services.

This allowed the government to claim that its economic policy was aimed at these objectives, and would therefore contribute more to improving the situation than would technological obstetrics. Finally, the economic consequences of increased ivnestment in maternity care were contested. The government costed the Short Report proposals at £160 million, not £25 million, and challenged the projected saving of £152 million on the grounds that preventable handicap had been overestimated initially. On all counts the government produced good arguments, largely based on allegedly 'progressive' ideas about health being determined by social circumstances, not medical care. The Conservatives used the arguments opportunistically, of course, for they were (and still are) unable to offer practical alternatives to improve social conditions or even develop medical services. The government's response to the Select Committee was a well-dressed argument covering a cost-cutting exercise. Its power derived from the clothes it borowed from its liberal opponents.

Once the territory of professionalism has been abandoned, political responses to it polarise into collaboration or confrontation. When it suits the sectional interests of organised labour, an alliance with the medical profession against the left is acceptable, justified by the cult of expertise. When it suits the interests of government, confrontation between organised labour and professional power can be utilised – as with the pay beds dispute in the mid-seventies – and even the most conservative trade union or Labour Party leader can be left-wing, for a while. Even when organised labour acted for the nation as a whole, in the 1945-50 administration, it was only able to create a temporary alliance between itself and the professionals running health care. As the value of collaboration declined, confrontation became the only tactic left.

For this reason the labour movement is losing its influence on the politics of health. Making decisions about priorities is accepted as an expert's affair, and the experts themselves are seen as untrustworthy and unreliable. Where Labour supporters retain influence, particularly after the Conservative purge of Health Authority chairs in 1982, they do so because their affiliations are no obstacle to acceptance of DHSS orthodoxy. Labour representatives on Health Authorities who actually promote public responses to change in health service provision are rare, often short-lived, birds. The polarisation between professionals and unionists, experts and the laity, facilitates Conservative control of health politics. Opposition to this or that cut or closure is pushed to the margins of political influence, where it can grow into opposition to *all* cuts and closures. Active opposition from outside the decision-making network helps those fostering defensive and insular attitudes and passivity in the face of cuts. The opportunities to present alternative strategies for development pass because no organised effort is made to cross the divide between professionalism and labour movement politics. As a conservative orthodoxy about NHS administration, finance and clinical activity sweeps all before it, the opposition adopts contrary stances, for lack of any other.

Switching Resources

Health economics is the best example of this polarity. On the left many feel that the prime problem of the NHS is a shortage of money. If we were to spend a larger proportion of our GDP on health care, we would resolve problems of low pay, poor facilities and inadequate technical services. A government boosting the NHS budget at the expense, say, of defence spending, could achieve twin objectives: the health service would be modernised, with renewed morale; and new work, and wealth, would be created in building and supply industries, and

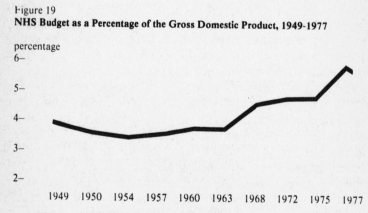

Figure 19
NHS Budget as a Percentage of the Gross Domestic Product, 1949-1977

Source: Royal Commission on the NHS, *Report*, 1979.

Figure 20
Spending on Hospitals and General Practitioner Services, 1949-1978

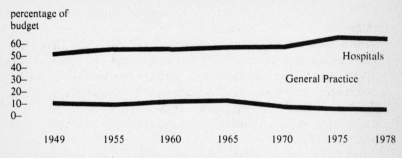

Source: Royal Commission on the NHS, *Report*, 1979.

Figure 21
Increases in Hospital Services, 1971-1977

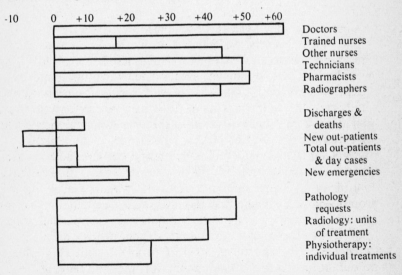

Source: S. Haywood and A. Alaszewski, *Crisis in the Health Service*, 1980.

in the NHS itself. As part of a short-term economic strategy for recovery from the monetarists' depression, this is sound enough. In the longer term, it may simply postpone the economic crisis in health care, and possibly permit another Conservative revival.

Britain, like other capitalist countries, has spent an increasing proportion of its GDP on health care, as Figure 19 shows.

Within this expenditure, however, a growing proportion has been devoted to hospital services, rather than community services, as is shown by Figure 20.

The output from this increased expenditure is difficult to measure. Real improvements in the duration and quality of life have been achieved, but they are hard to assess and all too often small-scale. Enormous efforts are necessaray for a low yield. 'Productivity', in terms of increased numbers of patients discharged from hospital, or seen for the first time in outpatient clinics, has not increased proportionally to the increased use of technology, nor to increased staff deployment, as illustrated in Figure 21.

An under-capitalised health care industry has deployed more and more workers to achieve disproportionately smaller growth in yield. If the volume of illness already known to the health service is only the tip of the iceberg of medical problems in the population, how much would it cost to uncover the hidden need by simply extending the present system?

Those defending the NHS may say that they do not want to extend the present service, but to change it. That may be true, even allowing for the different enthusiasm shown for change by Labour when in opposition and when in office. The problem in health care that reformers have to solve is the rising costs of limited success. Conservatism uses the slogan 'infinite demand, finite resources' to blame the population using the NHS for wanting 'a pill for every ill'. To reply that the reverse is true, and that we face finite demand with infinite resources, implies that control of demand and resources is within reach. Since professionals dominate decision-making over the use of resources, and are jealous of their autonomy, the onus lies with reformers to show how professionalism fits in with their plans for change. Conservatism has no problem with this; they encourage professional enthusiasm for the market-economy, and use professionals as mediators between the private and public health sectors. Socialists have great problems, however, for they generally have no alternative ethic of health care that makes sense to professional workers. Nursing can divide, unchecked by Labour movement initiatives, into a highly skilled workforce organised by the RCN and a less skilled group organised in trade unions. Medicine has been handed to the BMA, whilst rival professional bodies like the MPU have been retained as havens for doctors inclined towards the left. The Socialist Medical Association (now the Socialist Health Association) has its real base in the Labour Party, not in the health service, and so acts as an organiser of health workers already committed to Labour attitudes.

The Conservative slogan 'infinite demand, finite resources' is powerful because it is partly true. The political trick lies in not defining the origins of 'demand', and so implying that the fault lies with the consumers. We know that this is absurd, for demand in health care is a product of the market relationship between the customer and the tradesmen. It is the doctor who turns the wants of the patient into services – medicines, blood tests, operations, X-rays – that cost so much. Certainly the patient, as customer, can influence the doctor's decisions, but so too can the drug industry, the companies making scanners or analysers, and the manufacturers of scalpels, sutures and sterilisers. Few, if any, of those keen to teach us about 'infinite demand, finite resources', countenance serious action against commercial interests. (It was an exceptional Conservative Health Minister, Enoch Powell, who broke drug company price-fixing cartels in the early sixties, to reduce NHS drug spending). Nor is the Tory Party a front-runner in plans to reorganise the health professions, to make them accountable for what they do. Unfortunately, neither are their rivals.

Hopes persist that more and better management and planning will contain the 'infinite demand' of health professionals and their commercial sponsors for more and more resources. If economic recovery occurs, conventional planning and administrative methods may work enough to limit cost increases, but any subsequent economic decline would not stop health services eating more and more into GDP. When the public are the over-consuming villains, health spending can be limited by rationing services, and an undemocratic administrative structure can impose priorities in rationing. If we take the professionals and the supply industries as the source of infinite demand, what mechanisms can we use to constrain them? Having policies is easy for our resolutionary left. Lacking the means to enact them is the left's major weakness.

CHAPTER 9

A New Kind of Health Service?

If the Labour Party hopes to form a government in the 1980s or 1990s that can retain and develop a state-run health service without relying on the private sector, it must satisfy demands from three sources: the state, the population as a whole and the health professions. The state will be primarily concerned with getting value for money in health care, and secondly with satisfying the other two claimants. The population will want no less than it has had before, except, perhaps, for less medical interference in social issues (like fertility control), and will certainly want something new and worthwhile to justify changes required in the NHS. The professionals will demand that their privileges are retained or enlarged or that new advantages be offered in place of older privileges. Not only must the new government satisfy these demands, but also it must continue to satisfy them, repeatedly resolving the conflicts that will arise between the state, the people and the professionals. That may seem beyond the capabilities of the Labour Party and the labour movement generally, and in the short term we cannot expect dramatic progress. In the longer term, however, the prospects are much better, and the labour movement's strength much greater than it currently appears to be.

British 'socialism' is at its strongest when shaping the state, even when it shapes it in the interests of capital. Our starting-point for renewing National Health Service must be with state, and with most evolved political strategy for state health care available to the labour movement, the *Black Report* on inequalities in health. A reforming government connected to the NHS will have the advantage of an expansionary economic policy. Renewed investment in public spending will allow health services to be retained instead of cut, new jobs to be created in health care, and a start made on replacing ageing facilities with new ones. Health service expenditure will continue to rise, but probably at a faster rate. The government's objectives in NHS development must be determined by overall economic development, and a future Labour-controlled DHSS will need to apply constant restraints on health care spending, simply because of the general ability of health services to use all resources available to them. If the balance between productive and service industries within the national economy shifts back towards manufacturing industry, the proportion of GDP spent on the NHS can be increased, and health service expansion be used to create new service-industry jos. At some point in economic recovery, health care spending is likely to reach a plateau as it did in the seventies, and at that point the state's regulatory mechanisms for controlling health care will be tested. Demand for further expansion will not, and cannot, be reduced. The professional organisations will define need, in conjunction with the supply industries and public demand, just as they have done in the past.

Nationalisation of, say, the surgical supply industry will not necessarily resolve this problem, for such an industry amy be an important source of profits and employment and itself need to maximise output. The Hungarian pharmaceutical industry has played a leading role in the Hungarian 'economic miracle', by acting in collaboration with West German drug companies and promoting drug exports, particularly to the Third World, in a way comparable to the Western multinationals. Domestic consumption of medicines in Hungary has risen to the point where the government now seeks ways of restricting demand or at least transferring costs to the consumer.

This continuous expansion of demand from professionals and commercial suppliers is not simply due to new problems being manufactured by health professionals suffering from a lack of work, or industries anxious to maintain profit-rates. Surgeons trained to replace damaged heart valves may respond to the decreasing incidence of valve diseases by inventing new operations, of dubious value, but they do not account for much of the potential growth in medical care. Machines that monitor a baby's heart rate during its birth do more for their manufacturer's profits than for the baby (or its mother), but that does not undermine the usefulness of all obstetric technology. The dominant factor promoting change in medical techniques will be the changing pattern of disease. Problems will be tranformed, but not eradicated, by the combined impact of social change and improved health care. If efforts to reduce risk factors causing heart disease, or to detect malignant changes early enough for them to be treated, are effective, the present epidemics of these conditions will abate. Their decline will uncover a burden of degenerative diseases already well known – all the forms of arthritis, the different types of nervous system deterioration causing dementia, a range of disorders in our immune defence systems.

Health and Social Change

Continued social change will also create new problems. Prolonged mass unemployment seems likely to have adverse effects on both mental and physical health. Reduced working time, increased personal mobility and higher standards of education may produce negative as well as positive changes, with increased strain on social and family relationships and changed sexual attitudes and behaviour that provoke ill health rather than good health. The epidemic of genital herpes, said to be affecting 22 million Americans, is evidence that new health problems can arise on mass scale. The appearance of a new and often fatal disease, involving suppression of the body's immune defence system, amongst a largely homosexual population in New York and other American cities, demonstrates that medical technology and research have a sure future.

For the state, the problem will be one of finding an appropriate response to each problem. If long-term unemployment initially causes depression, family breakdown and an increased risk of suicide, and provokes outbreaks of heart disease and cancer at a later date, how should the state respond? Arguing that reductions in unemployment should be top priority for any government evades much of the problem. Those not rapidly re-absorbed into a re-exanded economy may become a reservoir of illness in the future, particularly if economic growth is slow, and full employment becomes unattainable for a decade or more. What resources should be deployed to meet the residual needs created by prolonged, mass unemployment? What are the best mechanisms for reducing demoralisation and depression, maintaining social and family relationships, and avoiding the utter hopelessness that precedes suicide?

A state concerned with getting value for money will need to work out its answers. If it does not, commercial and professional interests will produce apparently effective responses that are undoubtedly useful to themselves. The wider use of antidepressants, a rash of group psychotherapy clinics, and individual psychoanalysis on the NHS, may be useful responses, but may not be the most cost-effective way to cope with the new problems. The creation of unemployment centres, the deployment of councellors, or the massive expansion of adult education may have a much greater impact on the burden of ill health. For the state to make a choice between options, it will have to know more about the problems, and be more involved in the practicalities of their solution, than it has been in the past. A new kind of NHS will require, for its proper functioning, a new kind of state apparatus.

We have the elements of that kind of state, although they are not all incorporated in the Labour tradition. A broad perspective on health, taking into account the social origins of ill health, is the best part of our inheritance. We have a National Health Service more efficient *and* comprehensive than any health service outside socialist Europe, and we have plenty of ideas about social control methods drawn both from our own experience and from the wider experience of planned economies.

A government committed to planned health care would need a coherent, integrated programme of measures to improve the living standards of these social groups with the poorest health. These measures are the familiar elements of reform programmes: more jobs; more and better homes; better standards of education; higher benefits for the unemployed, the retired, the disabled and those at home caring for children or dependent adults. We can debate the qualities of assorted plans, but at least have the basic principles available to us. What we lack is a clear idea of how to finance this redistribution of wealth, given that current taxation seems to have reached its limits, and a clear idea of how to organise it all, given the postwar boom in clumsy bureaucracy and the growth of a benefits maze.

Adjusting the present tax system may be possible, and a future Labour government may try to 'squeeze the rich until the pips squeak', but its ability to stay in office may be weakened by such a policy, unless it has overwhelming popular support. In a taxation system that already hurts the relatively low-paid considerably, how much lasting popular support can be generated by a swingeing attack on the super-rich? How many in middle income brackets could be made nervous at the prospect of being the next victims? Would the finance generated be enough to pay for the redistribution programme, or would it need supplementation? Taxes on consumer goods may be an extra source of finance, but are equally risky. They may be both unpopular and also contribute to patterns of illness. If the income from taxation on smoking is important to the Exchequer, then taxation levels must not be so high that they inhibit consumption to the point where Exchequer income drops. Without heavy taxation, cigarette consumption will remain a mass habit, even if it declines over several generations, and will generate its own burden of illness requiring responses from the health service. As we approach the limits of the taxation system, only two options remain. The objective of wealth redistribution can be abandoned, or a new mechanism established – for the control of the accumulation of wealth.

The Role of the State

Organising social change on this scale is another issue, but it has an impact on health service structure. Within the labour movement there is a polarised argument over national versus local government control of health care. The centralist view, supporting a nationally-controlled NHS run by a more open version of the present command structure, fits with the Fabian, managerial tradition in Labour thinking. Its advocates point to the advantages of centralism: the imposition of standards of service in areas where dominant political interests would otherwise veto them; the potential for planned allocation of resources according to need; the opportunities for containing costs and running an efficient service. If health care were open to local government control, Conservative areas would run different, and probably inferior, services than Labour-controlled areas, despite being richer. The post war experience of local control of, and therefore local variation within, public housing and education would simply be extended into health services. To prevent such variation, a centralised control structure should be retained so that local governments in the 'wrong' hands could always be circumvented when it came to providing health care.

The opposite, devolutionist, view bases its arguments in favour of local government control on the measurement of need and the co-ordination of services. Who can best judge the needs of a locality, if not the elected representatives of that locality?

Electoral democracy allows public understanding and expectations to be married to health service necessities, so that what the people want and what they appear to need can be considered, at least in principle. Since health is closely related to housing and education, should it not also have the same controlling structure, so that health priorities can really influence housing policy and the content of education?

Neither argument will help us in the future, for both derive from the past circumstances of the labour movement. The centralist strand of Labour thinking demonstrated its strengths and weaknesses during the postwar boom, shaping the mixed economy and the Welfare State but without correcting variations in the quantity and quality of health care between regions and classes. Planning in health care is in its infancy, and to grow this requries an economic recovery comparable to the postwar boom. Our industrial base has declined so far, and our role as a nation become so peripheral, that such an economic recovery seems unlikely. Regional variations in the provision of health care seem likely to increase, not decrease, as an increasing share of health care passes into private hands. Conservatism actively promotes this public-private mix, and uses the existing centralised control structure to enforce a version of devolution, fostering local Health Authorities that reflect commercial and professional interests more closely than ever. Labour's centralists can try to borrow the right's slogan, 'patients before politics', to justify their idea of a command structure that allocates according to *need*, but if they do so they leave the right to organise *wants*.

The devolutionist position has an honourable origin in municipal socialism, but a dishonourable place in both public and professional perceptions. Local government is based on passive democracy, in which competition between interest groups determines policy choices. Labour's contribution to local government has too often been to encourage passivity and foster a corrupting system of patronage, matching the Old Boy network of Conservatives, ratepayers and Chamber of Commerce. Enthusiasm for control of health services by local politicians does not seem great within the working class, whilst health professionals usually regard it with horror and quote their experience of Social Services departments as a warning against municipal control. A new breed of Labour councillors may change all that, but they will first have to survive a Conservative

attack on local government powers, and then show that
municipal politics can be reformed, before local government
control of health services becomes possible.

From the state's viewpoint, the structure of the NHS will need
changing to permit the state's objectives to be realised. A new
Labour administration that rebuilds the public sector as the
skeleton of the economy and the society will aim to develop a
streamlined and efficient health service that provides a
comprehensive service. It will have to accept a range of over-
riding objectives that it must pursue, even if that provokes
conflict. The first objective will be to control demand for health
services, particularly the demand prompted by commercial
interests. The second will be to respond to unmet needs, which
will have to be sought out and measured. A third objective will
be the creation of a flexible structure, open to future change.
Finally, a renewed National Health Service will need to become
cost-effective, through continued measurement of the outcome
of its activity.

Nationalising the Drug Companies

Controlling demand will require restrictions on professional
activities, constraints on commercial involvement in health care,
and modification of public expectations. The left advocates
nationalisation of the pharmaceutical industry, and could also
reasonably include the surgical supply companies feeding the
NHS. Whilst this may help constrain commercial pressure on
the NHS, through direct government intervention,
nationalisation alone does not guarantee adequate control over
exceesive drugs costs. State companies obey economic laws, and
surplus value will be in demand, so extra mechanisms for
restricting drug and equipment consumption will be necessary.
These restrictions could be applied without public control of the
supply industries, but evasion of controls had developed into a
fine art within the drugs industry in particular. Tight control
over expenditure on promotion of new products, replacement of
company representatives with unbiased technical advisors, and
subsidies for scientific publications are all in the labour
movement's armoury, awaiting application. The case for
nationalising the pharmaceutical industry is, therefore a
particularly strong one; indeed, a drug industry answerable to
public not private interests is essential to a health service which

has an upper limit on its spending.

The problem for the labour movement, and for a reforming government, will arise in the timing of changes. Reductions in drug consumption will mean closures of industrial plant, even if only in the packing industry that processes German, American or Swiss medicines, and that will jeopardise jobs. Workers in pharmaceutical companies may be opposed to nationalisation plans that threaten their industry, just as many tobacco workers tend to dismiss the evidence linking cigarettes to cancer as 'lies, damned lies and statistics'. One union with a substantial membership in the drugs industry, ASTMS, is distinctly cool about public ownership, and the Labour Party advocates the nationalisation of only one major drug company, and the extension of controlling regulations over others. This may make good political sense within the trade union movement, particularly during a recession, but it contributes little to controlling the production of wealth, and only a little more to economic restraint within health care. If there is an answer to this problem, it will lie with forward planning of ecnomomic change, retraining for new work, and the development of alternative products or alternative industries. None of that can come quickly, in the form of dramatic, revolutionary change. Nor do we need to wait for a new kind of Labour government to be formed, before changes begin. On the contrary, unless it can show that it has realistic methods for implementing its programme, Labour seems unlikely to win the overwhelming support it needs.

Controlling the Professionals

Public control over the drug and surgical supply industries will have an impact on professional activity, but only influence one of the factors determining demand. The role of professionals in their market relationships will also need controls applied to it, even though that may prove politically perilous. There is a constant contradiction between professionalism (as it now stands) and public service, and this could grow as the government emphasises public service at the expense of professional power.

A Labour government will need to challenge (continually) the validity of professional activity, from the state's cost-effectiveness viewpoint. Are the things that professionals do worthwhile? Has the proposal for a new service nationwide, been tested with pilot studies, or is it being promoted for other reasons? Are particular clinical activities being neglected, even though they would almost certainly be useful and effective, whilst less useful practices are continued? If the National Health Service had been subject to this kind of interrogation in the sixties and seventies, coronary care units may not have developed at the rate they did, at such cost, and to so little effect. Monitoring of labour and childbirth might not have become so fashionable, so fast, that inexperienced staff misused unfamiliar techniques and machines, and mismanaged the labour of so many women. On the other hand, we might have more facilities for kidney dialysis and kidney transplantation, and perhaps a community-based programme to combat heart disease and high blood pressure.

To influence the application of health sciences in this way, we will need more than a strong DHSS that controls the distribution of resources. The local use of resources, the choice of options, demands a local challenge to the alliance of professional and commercial interests, from knowledgeable and articulate public bodies. For trade unions, Community Health Councils, ethnic minority groups or women's movement organisations to be knowledgeable and articulate on professional and technical issues they will need to be confident that experts do not always know best, and have the support of at least some of those experts themselves. The labour movement's own expertise, in the MPU and the SHA, may have been weakened by thirty years of pragmatism, but it is not beyond recovery. The women's movement has done more than any other political force to demonstrate the power of alliances between professionals and the laity, particularly around the defence of the 1967 Abortion Act. Just as preparatory changes are needed in economic strategy and trades union industrial perspective, so the beginnings of alliances between professionals and public organisations must appear before fundamental change can occur within the NHS.

Health Education

When Conservative politicians talk about controlling the demand for health care, they almost always mean stopping an ignorant but greedy population from using the NHS too much.

Demand for private medical care, on the other hand, is evidence of needs cruelly ignored by an insensitive state, and is to be encouraged. Since all change exacts a price from someone somewhere, the users of the health service must pay the price for its 'excessive' costs, and learn to forfeit the service and look after themselves. Yet health education has never been very significant to the NHS, and at first sight this seems puzzling. If people expect too much from the NHS, and use it unnecessarily, why does the state not educate the population into self-reliance? If the English and Scottish Health Education Councils had a combined budget of £4 million pounds in 1977-78 compared with hospital running costs of £4,736 million, was the government seriously doing anything to control public demand? It is tempting to see the underfunding of health education as a terrible failure on the part of government, a sign of the state's shortsightedness and stupidity. More money spent on health education would reduce demand for health care, and resources would be freed for the needy. That is an illusion. Successive governments have neglected health education deliberately, so that public demand for health services could be more easily controlled, by minimising it.

The idea that the needy, in medical terms, are only a small proportion of those using the NHS, is as untrue as the belief that the health service meets all needs. What health service users need, and what they actually get, may be different, but that is not entirely their fault and certainly does not negate their need. What people may need, to preserve their health, may not be dealt with at all by the NHS. They constitute the submerged portion of the iceberg of clinical need. Health education, to be effective, should encourage appropriate use of services by those in need, and may well increase demand for health care rather than reduce it. The more women think in terms of future risks of cervical cancer, the more will use screening services for early detection of malignant changes in the cervix. An individual suffering from recurrent headaches or backaches caused by prolonged unresolved stresses at work or in personal relationships, may consume pain-killers bought over the counter, pursue brain tumours or spinal arthritis with all the technology available, or take up an offer of counselling that ultimately resolves the background problems. Each option reflects a different level of understanding of the symptoms and their origins, and leads to a different kind of health expenditure.

Which option is the cheapest depends on the quantity of pain-killers eventually taken, the number of out-patient attendances and investigations, and the cost of employing a counsellor or clinical psychologist for the necessary time. The successful treatment, reflecting the highest level of understanding, could easily be the most expensive. Health education could then increase NHS spending, rather than reduce it.

For this reason health education has received a low priority in government spending. Much health education is instructive, either telling us not to do things that others suggest are worthwhile (like smoking cigarettes, or drinking and driving), or encouraging a consumer orientation towards a better diet, more exercise and healthier personal habits. This approach is designed to counter the positively harmful pressures that undermine public health – the active promotion of tobacco and alcohol consumption, for example. Health education of this kind demonstrates the state's concern for health conservation, and supports its claims of impotance in the face of market needs and human nature. It allows governments and harassed professionals alike to blame people for their ignorance in rejecting advice. A government warning on a cigarette packet is expected to outweigh the relief, pleasure and status provided by tobacco. The techniques of health educationalists are not to blame; the dishonesty and hypocrisy belong to successive governments that have tolerated health hazards and made only token responses to them.

Missing from the range of health education initiatives are the potentially expensive ones. No comprehensive advisory service routinely assesses health hazards in the built environment or at the workplace, from the viewpoint of the resident or the worker respectively. The number of adults who have been offered personal advice on their health and its maintenance, based on their family's health, their own past experience of illness, their occupation and their current physical state, is very small indeed. Health visitors have such an advisory role, and their numbers have increased (from 6,400 in 1967 to 10,250 a decade later), but their major preoccupation is child-care, and other problems take second place. General practitioners may be able to provide such a service, but there is little evidence that they do so, even when asked. Finally, until 1974 no mechanism existed to actively promote an understanding of health policies within the population. The Community Health Councils can perform that task, but they are not obliged to, and may even be at risk of administrative reprisals if they adopt too political a stance. A government that seeks to maintain the population's health and take all realistic measures to prevent illness and injury will need to fill these gaps, if it is serious about health education. In doing so, it will not be able to argue that it will reduce demand for medical care, and therefore must be very sure that other regulatory mechanisms work well.

Controlling the Carers

The regulatory mechanisms have one over-riding purpose. They should allow need for health care to be met effectively and efficiently, as cheaply as possible. Effectiveness and efficiency cannot be judged unless the scope of illness and disability is known, and the impact of health care measured. Some types of need are well studied, and medical intervention is sometimes carefully analysed for its faults and virtues, but there are surprising gaps in our knowledge and our actions. The Confidential Enquiries into Maternal and Perinatal Deaths are useful, retrospective reviews of the causes of death of mothers and babies in childbirth, but we have no accurate data on the numbers of handicapped babies born, or on the causes of their handicaps. Tonsils are no longer removed as readily as they once were, because tonsillectomy has been shown to be unnecessary in most instances, and positively dangerous in some. Mastectomy has not been shown to be any better a treatment for most breast cancers than alternative techniques like removal of only the tumour (plus radiotherapy), yet mastectomies are performed routinely. Nor is economic value always used to monitor, and influence, health care provision, despite the managerialist approach to health service administration.

The ways in which general practitioenrs prescribe drugs are monitored, at a central pricing office, and each GP is informed of his or her relative cost to the NHS, compared with other GPs in the same area and nationally. If a doctor's prescribing is markedly higher than the average for his or her area, a DHSS Regional Medical Officer can visit him or her and discuss use of medicines. In England, in the seventies, about 10% of GPs had prescribing costs 25% or more above the average for their locality, but only 7% were visited. In theory, persistent excessive prescribing can be punished by deductions from payments to the overprescribing doctor. This is a rare event. The Royal Commission on the NHS, reporting in 1979, noted that no GPs in England had been 'fined' since 1972.

This demonstrates one problem in pursuing effectiveness and efficiency. Measurement of services, and of their impact and value, is possible, but it is not useful unless it leads on to changes in activity. The mechanisms of measurement, and even for initiating change, exist, but the cult of expertise inhibits their use. Tonsillectomy can become a less common operation, when Ear, Nose and Throat surgeons accept that it is no longer necessary on a mass scale. Mastectomy, on the other hand, remains a comonplace surgical procedure, despite doubts about its overall value, because general surgeons do not yet accept that alternative approaches can be equally good (or bad), and less disfiguring. Doctors who over-prescribe are rarely penalised because penalties would provoke a conflict on terms favourable to professionalism, and few administrators have the confidence to pick such a fight. The regulatory mechanisms that will be needed to resist professional and commercial demands for increased funding will have an additional function. They will permit wider, more detailed and more accurate measurement of the work done by health professionals, and the consequences of this work for those in need. They will also direct attention towards unmet need, and away from over-treated demand. Although both professionals and public will be encouraged by the right to see tighter management of health care as stifling and constricting, its real importance will be in the impetus it gives to change.

Long Term Changes in Health Care

The ability to change, and the incorporation of flexibility as a management principle into health care, cannot be left out of our thinking for the NHS. State-run health care has passed through several stages of evolution, each lasting about forty years, with the most recent phases ending with a major change in the provision of services. From 1830 to 1870 the state's concern was with legislation to protect health, and provision of help was left to families, charities and the parish. From about 1870 onwards, social provision of sickness benefits became the dominant issue, and the state played only a minor role until the first great turning point, in 1911. Between the National Insurance Act and the foundation of the NHS, the control of the major infectious diseases became possible, and popular demands shifted target from general practitioner services to specialist attention and hospitals beds.

The NHS opened up health care to the population, and gave curative medicine its greatest impetus to date. The architects of future changes in health services need to remember the step-wise development of medical care, and plan for *two* turning-points: the imminent point, somewhere in the eighties or nineties; and the next one! If we enter a period in which state responsibilities diminish, and market powers increase, the subsequent phase may apply corrective, controlling methods to the market and to professionalism that we would consider unthinkable now. If, on the other hand, the NHS changes emphasis towards preventive and community-based care in the coming decades, we may have to face a spectrum of health problems in the first quarter of the 21st century that we can barely understand now.

What kind of health service can meet all these criteria? What mechanism offers efficiency, effectiveness and flexibility, provides a comprehensive service, and aims at needs rather than at wants? Only the military model, which inspired planners after both world wars, and which allowed Britain to retain its hierarchy of generalist and specialist services, despite the specialist domination of scientific advances. The military model presupposes that services are needed, and seeks out need instead of waiting for demand. It requires its personnel with the widest skills to be up at the front, close to the action, near to the need. They decide on priorities, and pass difficult or even insoluble problems to more distant resources staffed by personnel with narrower, more specialised, skills. They in turn can use a third resource, designed to provide long-term care and support to those needing it. Our health service matches this model, in its three tiers of generalists, specialist and long-term care, but it has grown in an uneven way. Resources have been requisitioned by the second tier (the hospitals services) in a way that has threatened to undermine the whole structure. Both the front line and the long-stay institutions have been relatively neglected, and as a consequence the whole mechanism is jeopardised. A forward-looking government will have little choice but to strengthen the crucial front-line, or abandon the model altogether. The former choice is a development of the existing situation, and requires no dramatic change. The latter option, expressed as a renaissance of private medicine, is perfectly possible, but requires the present structure to be dismantled.

If hospital services and staff begin to work in community settings, the military model will have a second lease of life. If general practitioners with interests in private medicine cooperate in building new private hospitals and clinics, in which they can dabble in their specialist interest, the hierarchic structure of the NHS will be undermined. The choice made will be determined, in part, by the responses of the public and the professionals to the options available. The state, when concerned with meeting need, must favour the military model. When it rejects needs as important criteria, and concentrates instead on the renewal of profitability, the military model becomes superfluous. Market forces stress that public demand and professional enthusiasm can fruitfully combine, in private medicine. Can the left perceive a comparable coincidence of public and professional interests, around policies and practices genuinely concerned with people's needs?

The Black Report

The nearest we have come to such a perception, as yet, is expressed in the *Black Report* on inequalities in health. This report is often seen primarily as a compendium of facts about class and health, and its political, programmatic, content is neglected. Yet it breaks with significant labour movement traditions without losing its overall Fabian character, and for that reason alone can be described as the most significant single document on health since the Beveridge Report.

The *Black Report* takes a broad perspective, combining an anti-poverty programme with proposals for purposive, planned health care initiatives. The anti-poverty programme has two remarkable elements in it: it argues that reduction in wealth differentials must be a necessary part of any attempt to improve living standards; and that education should be aimed at 'autonomy', the reclaiming of power by individuals, from the state. Reducing wealth differentials means limiting the highest income, and has implications for the medical profession – particularly for that élite group of consultants with merit awards and large private practices. Limitation of income through a ceiling on earnings is a frontal attack on the accumulation of wealth, and is incompatible with the private pursuit of profit. Education for 'autonomy' can be seen as a challenge to professionalism's dominant expression, for such autononmy would require sharing of the secrets and skills that define professionalism, and that allow it a special place in the market. And the return of power, from state to citizen, suggests that the state can be used by citizens, instead of it using them – an experience only shared by the most powerful, privileged and wealthy in Britain today.

The proposals for the health service are similarly significant. The *Black Report* argues that only through the development of community-based services, at the expense of growth in the hospital sector, can we hope to meet needs for medical care. It argues for effective action to reduce cigarette smoking, listing detailed measures to cut cigarette advertising and improve health education. It advocates a national Health Development Council, that will review the health implications of all government policy. It outlines priorities in health care, arguing for special emphasis on the needs of children, mothers, the disabled and the elderly, and proposing District Health Programmes based on these priorities. The Report suggests that ten areas of great social need should be the targets for special health care programmes, aimed at measuring needs and evolving services to meet them. And it breaks new ground by concentrating on work hazards, and the need to investigate, study, and react to, health risks within industry and commerce.

Armed with its programe, the Report falters. Health professionals are encouraged to accept their responsibilities for meeting need, and the pharmaceutical industry is countered by piecemeal measures like generic substitution. The Black Committee could not resolve all problems, of course, and therefore stayed on the familiar ground of legislation, social planning and centralised organisation. Like so many reformers before, it drew back from the potential danger of conflict with professional and commercial interests. That is political territory, to be contested by politicians with professional or popular backing.

CHAPTER 10

Patients and Politics

Could health professionals support the kind of programme promoted by the *Black Report*? Would strengthening the military model of health care provision be supported or resisted by those who would operate it? To predict professional responses we must know both the balance of gain and loss, for professional workers, in changing the emphasis of the NHS, and also the balance of political influence within the professions themselves.

The gains for professionals would include an expansion in numbers and a change in roles or status. If the objective of a reformed health service is to prevent as much ill health as possible, and its methods require close contact with the population, there must be an increase in staffing levels. In some places this increase may be dramatic, because present services are minimal or non-existent. The TUC estimated in the late seventies that one in three workers had no access to any kind of health care at their workplace. Yet the workplace is both a source of health hazards, and a point at which health services can reach the sections of the population facing the greatest health risks. Extension of the health service into industry and commerce would have to occur if the government were serious in its policy on health, and could involve more than first-aid responses to industrial injury. Workplace screening for high-blood pressure, cervical cancer, or signs of heart or lung disease would be possible, and could offer basic methods of health conservation to those least likely to receive them through usual NHS channels. Assessments of risks within the workplace may be a managerial or trade union responsibility, but it is hampered the dearth of advice and information available to trade unionists, and the resistance of both management and, in some cases, the workforce, to investigations that may threaten profitability. An industrial health service, growing through the combination of existing industrial medical departments, the Employment Medical Advisory Service, trade union health and safety representatives, and backed by legislative powers and responsibilities, could become a major instrument in the new health policy.

Expanding Primary Care

Expansion of other community-based services may not be so great as in industry, but it would be no less necessary. If education about health and illness is seen as the basis for better health care, the number of educators must increase. Ten thousand health visitors can barely satisfy statutory requirements for care of the under-fives at the moment. Enlarging their role, to include advice and support for the elderly, or specialist education for those with long-term illnesses, requires their profession to expand as well. If the NHS is to move away from false solutions, like the endless use of tranquillisers, to more lasting and real solutions to personal and social problems, we will need a supply of skilled staff who will replace the profitable drugs and tonics promoted by the pharmaceutical industry. We already have some of these workers, but only in small numbers. Counsellors, clinical psychologists and psychotherapists work within the NHS, but as specialists often subordinate or ancillary to medicine. Elevated to a front-line role, they would need to adopt a more combative style, perhaps working with groups of people more than they do now, and advising other health workers about resolving the painful problems of illness, death and bereavement, whilst still retaining personal and individual relationships with their patients. The same applies to physiotherapists, nurses and occupational therapists, whose work within individuals' homes and in group settings could not be the same as it is now in the hospitals and long-stay institutions of the NHS.

The expansion of the front-line, of primary care, could only work through changes in professional roles. The idea that the medical profession in general practice could mimic its specialist equivalents in the hospitals, by evolving a network of subordinate workers directed by the central figure, the doctor, appeals to medical vanity but not to realism. General practitioners as a whole have not attempted to deal with the need for medical care, except through responding to demand as best they can. Medical responses have been incomplete even then, prompting the development of alternative services based on the hospital network – the accident and emergency departments, massive out-patient clinics and walk-in psychiatric and child-care clinics that are such a feature of urban areas. Even the organisation of limited teams of support workers in general practice, primarily concerned with administrative rather than clinical work, has proceeded slowly. The idea that 'primary care teams' in a health service committed to meeting people's needs could be led by general practitioners owes its persistence to medical pride and complacency. Real changes in professional relationships would occur if primary care were made into the foundation of the NHS, and most of the benefit from such changes would go to non-medical professionals. Instead of general practitioners becoming like consultants, with empires of underlings, nurses, midwives, health visitors and other professional workers would gain some of the responsibilities and autonomy currently enjoyed by doctors, dentists, opticians and pharmacists. Unlike this latter group, the new primary care professionals will work within the constraints of a health service with national and local objectives. For the NHS, the greatest professional problem will be integrating the independent contractor professions into planned primary care services, and not the evolution of a leading role for general practitioners.

If planned primary care redefines professional roles, and boosts the numbers and status of subordinate professions, it also offers something to the specialist workers in the second line, the hospitals. The stronger the front-line, the more effective it is as a selective barrier to specialist care, the more specialist workers will support it. If antenatal clinics are packed 'cattle markets', giving brief and uninformative attention to large numbers of women with straightforward pregnancies, specialist skills become diluted and ineffective. If, on the other hand, routine antenatal care is devolved to midwives and doctors working near (or even at) the woman's home or workplace, specialist skills can be concentrated on those individual's whose pregnancies become complicated. The quality of specialist care depends on its concentration on appropriate problems, and the purpose of the front-line in the military model of health care is to select those problems accurately. For the specialist, then, the quality and quantity of primary care are crucial issues, for they determine the character of specialist services.

Flashpoints

Problems will arise within the hospital sector when expanding of primary care competes with hospital services for a greater share of resources, and when the hospital specialists' escape route into private medicine is closed, or even narrowed. New technological developments, now at the launch stage, will soon be promoted in a way that could harm as much as help in health care. One new technique, called nuclear magnetic resonance (NMR), measures the responses of body tissues to a magnetic field and allows magnetic maps of the body to be made. These maps can distinguish between normal and malignant tissue, give high-quality pictures of soft structures like muscle, internal organs and skin, and therefore have great diagnostic potential. A new range of NMR machines may follow 'computerised tomography' (CT scanners) into NHS hospitals, eating into health authority capital and current budgets and creating new professional skills before the real value of this improved diagnostic technique is measured. By the time that it is accepted that better diagnosis is little help unless better treatment is available, the machinery will be in place, and a second generation may be on order. Alternative approaches, perhaps involving long-term screening of hormone production in apparently healthy people, may predict those who will later develop malignancies *and* offer clues about different treatments, but will be pursued slowly because they have so little commercial value. The clamour for the new technology will be intense; the problem for the new NHS will be one of refusing to accept the rate of change dictated by an alliance of commercial and professional pressures.

Not all the problems will be so clear-cut. Microtechnology applied to human metabolism may make much of the present work of medical laboratories redundant, by taking the diagnostic processes to the individual under investigation. Small-scale, easily-operated machinery used on the hospital ward, in the local clinic, or within the home could cope with the diagnostic tests now done routinely, and on a mass scale, in centralised departments. If laboratory technicians are already becomine machine-minders, they may find themselves without machines to mind in the relatively near future. Health service administrators will come under pressure to reduce the number of laboratory technical staff, from all those who covet the money spent on them. Trade unions representing these workers will have to decide their priorities: to resist the new technology, to aim for the devolution of staff to decentralised facilities, or to develop some kind of Hospital Scientific Service, as a new collective expression for a dwindling workforce?

Restrictions on spending in NHS hospitals can be tolerated, at least by some professions, provided that there is an outlet for their ambitions in the private sector. What will happen if that outlet is reduced, or completely blocked? A reforming government could use a simple argument; all our resources are needed for the National Heath Service. If there is to be any private sector in health care, it can only be acceptable as a subcontractor to the NHS, like charitable abortion services or private nursing homes. The small private hospitals, and, more importantly, the administrative and clinical staff they have poached, will be needed for NHS work, according to NHS priorities, and will be drawn into public ownership.

The logic is sound, and such a policy should be pursued, but with three qualifications. The first is that expansion must be seen to be occurring, and its benefits must be felt by professions in health care as well as by the public. When most are experiencing the rewards of cooperation, they will be more likely to see the self-interest of private medicine for what it is, and that may be crucial to political development. The second is that some privately-owned services may be retained in a contracted-out relationship to the public service. It may do more harm than good to bring the charitable abortion agencies under NHS control, even if the take-over promised to increase their resources, since it would also expose them to the potentially unfavourable climate of professional politics. Debate, and conflict, about priorities in health care will not clarify issues instantly, and the balance between public and professional/commercial power inside the NHS will take time to change. Until then, there may be a good argument for keeping subordinate, privately-controlled services independent of the NHS proper. The same must inevitably apply, for a period of time, to the present independent contractor professions, for not all of them are likely to accept NHS inducements and instantly become salaried employees.

The final qualification is that serious attempt should be made to undermine the *principle* of private medicine, as a 'right' of suppliers and users alike. The qualification is a tactical one, but it has strategic implications as well. The new NHS will need the active cooperation of most of its present workforce, and the enthusiasm of new recruits. Whilst the balance of power may shift, no single group of workers can be disenfranchised without the risk of conflict that could damage the service. The more powerful the group, the more likely it is to resist a reduction in its power, and more damaging the conflict will be. Changing the emphasis in health care, re-allocating resources, and making decision-making a public as much as a professional responsibility, are assaults on the status quo that will need careful coordination.

The right will want an issue that will unite professional workers against the government, and 'professional freedom' will be its issue of choice. If NHS resources are expanding, and there is no overall erosion of professional incomes, the only aspect of professional freedom left is its 'liberal', market origins. The defence of private medicine may become the symbolic banner for a much wider reaction against declining powers. It is up to the left to prevent professional unity developing around such issues, by avoiding a battle on principles and sticking to concrete (and divisive) issues of resources and their use.

The Labour Party has a tradition of making tactical alliances in health politics, and that may give it the flexibility to control development. Unfortunately, it also has a second, and more recent, tradition of rejecting such alliances, when doing so provides short-term advantages. Labour in government may need a diversion if the problems of low pay remain insoluble, and the priviledges of wallet-conscious specialists are an admirable target, a counter-irritation, for angry trade unionists. Politicians may need to establish left-wing credentials within the labour movement, and confrontational politics can give them an opportunity to prove their militancy whilst screening much deeper compromises over power. The temptations are great, and will be amplified, behind the scenes, by professional and commercial interests. Alternative alliances, aimed at changing the balance of power, will be possible if serious efforts are made to develop collectivist ideas about public service within professional groups, and professional attitudes within trade unions, but such developments must exclude traditional conflicts on issue of 'principle'.

Scenarios

The disadvantages to health professionals from an expansion of primary care arise when planning of services clashes with professional autonomy. For professional groups like health visitors that are accustomed to goal-oriented activity and meeting statutory obligations, the conflicts may be minor. For those groups without a tradition of forward planning, measurement of outcome or even cooperation, the conflicts are likely to be prolonged and painful. The new NHS will demand accountability and collaborative efforts towards agreed objectives, and will offer better working conditions (through increased staffing) and more opportunities for the appropriate use of skills. Whether the advantages outweigh the disadvantages, and prevent a rebellion of the tradesmen, will depend on the political pressures constraining traditional professionalism. If the new primary care professions accept the necessary changes, the hospital specialists support them, and the population responds to them, the shopkeeper tradition in medicine, dentistry and pharmacy will be isolated and overcome. If the population is indifferent, other health professionals suspicious or hostile, and the hospital services neutral, traditional professionalism backed by commercial resources and right-wing politicians will take the initiative and block reform.

The best outcome would be when health workers and significant groups of the population both benefit from changes in approach and organisation, and were seen to benefit by the professionals opposing change, and by the general public. An expansion in staff numbers, coupled with the development of new facilities, would allow the caseloads of health professionals to shrink, and the work itself to spread across a wider range of skills. The appearance of more generalist workers, like health visitors and nurses, would fill the present gaps in the service and relieve the pressure on existing staff, whilst the introduction of more specialist staff, the psychologists, physiotherapists or chiropodists, would permit more in-depth care. Administrative tasks now done badly by clinical workers would devolve to administrative staff, so that even the potentially painful assessment of work done and not done could become the job of a specialist working alongside clinical staff. The responses from the people needing NHS services should act as catalysts to further change. More time will be available, and that alone should prove popular. Those looking after the elderly infirm, the physically and mentally handicapped, the mentally ill and the demented, will have highest priority in community services, and receive more help and support than before. Those working in industry and commerce will have access to new occupational health services that offer both personal screening and help with health hazards in the industrial environment. New approaches to health and the prevention of illness, and more personal attention for those with long-term disorders like arthritis, schizophrenia or epilepsy, would become possible as caseloads fell and contacts between health workers and service-users lengthened.

If the mutual benefits of change were re-inforced by publicity, and by more imaginative, down-to-earth health education in the media, the negative effects of changes could become tolerable for most health professionals. Reduced access to private medicine may anger some doctors and nurses, and some of their patients too, but a reduced market would still exist for them, and their reaction would be diluted by the positive responses of those benefiting from NHS expansion.

The right would try to organise resistance, and the BMA and the RCN might attempt to orchestrate resignations as the changes accelerated and private practice was eroded. If the government called the right's bluff, most professionals would vote with their feet, accepting the benefits of change and rejecting their own professional organisations' political advice. The right would have to judge its tactical moves carefully. Would a campaign to preserve private medicine be turned, by the media, into a campaign against new developments in health care, and would the professions be split rather than united? Would the trade unions take advantage of this potential split to project their own claims to be guardians of health care and true advocates of public services? And even if the pharmaceutical industry was still largely privately owned, would it be keen to risk its status by backing professionals campaigning against the public good, in defence of their own narrow interests? The most powerful professional group, the BMA, has only won conflicts over private medicine by its threats of retaliation against reforming governments. Its only attempt at direct industrial action in defence of private medicine, in 1975-6, was poorly supported by BMA members, and there is little reason for believing that the BMA, or any other professional group, could withstand a direct confrontation on unfavourable ground.

The political prognosis for health care could worsen, however, if a conflict between professionals and government (or trade unionists acting as proxy for government) occurs on ground favourable to the right. If the hospital consultants rebel against restrictions on private medicine, they may provoke a counter-move from the left that seeks to increase the restrictions. Perhaps a Private Members Bill aimed at 'strengthening' government legislation on part-time consultant contracts, tax liabilities on private health insurance, or nationalisation of private hospitals, could act as a focus for campaigns on the left and the right. Pressures for 'bans' on private medicine, expressed by demonstrations, pickets and eyeball-to-eyeball clashes at hospital gates, would also help organise the professional unity so desperately needed by the right.

The conflict over private medicine would become the dominant issue in health politics, eclipsing the effects of service expansion, and allowing professional organisations to launch their campaigns in defence of professional freedom. Surgeries, pharmacies and dentists' offices would become the local bases for an assault on the new reforms, and Britain could follow Chile (in 1972-3) and France (in 1981-2) as professional workers spearhead right-wing counter-offensives. The private sector would take advantage of the conflict to promote itself as a stable source of medicine in an otherwise chaotic system of health care. International drug monopolies could be tempted to join in, threatening precipitate closure of British-based concerns or economic retaliation for planned nationalisation, whilst the UK chemical industry sat on its hands and waited for the government to fall or back-down. Retreat would be the only realistic option for a government that had only just initiated its reform programme, and that did not have the power or backing to impose its policies on its opponents by direct force. The choices for action would be polarised once again, with loud voices advocating compromises in the style of the Wilson-Callaghan administration, and a minority shouting for more civil conflict. Each would become a replay of past efforts, the dogmatic imposition of old doctrines of 'mixed economy' or 'social revolution' on new circumstances, and each would pass the political initiative to the right.

Participatory Democracy

The responses of the population will make or break the new approach to health care. For the reforming government, the greatest problem will be the creation of mechanisms that encourage the coincidence of wants and needs. Since what each person needs, in medical terms, can only be known by asking him or her, the state will need some way of influencing the dialogue between the user and the provider of services. At the moment the relationships may be three-sided, between doctor, patient, and drug company, or health visitor, parent and milk manufacturer. The third, commercial side is physically absent from the dialogue, yet influences each party. How will the NHS replace the commercial interests with its own, cost-effective interests, in the daily encounters between health workers and their patients?

The answers could be that better education for all, and a tighter grip on drug firms and supply industries, would alter the relationship between professional and patient. So they might, but better education is more likely to increase demand than decrease it, and commercial evasion of regulations has not proved difficult so far. Nor are people likely to work up great enthusiasm for distant and long-term policies, when immediate political conflicts between the government and the pharmaceutical industry or the medical profession dominate the news bulletins. Strategies that give the population a passive role in changing and controlling health care leave people in the market-place, open to manipulation as consumers of goods. Alternative strategies, based on the involvement of people in making and carrying out decisions, may be more difficult to implement, and outside between individual, professional and state interests in health care. They depend on the mutual recognition of the problems and possibilities faced by the sick

individuals, professionals in health care, and the NHS as part of
the state. Such recognition comes through acceptance of
responsibility, rather than through more passive learning. This
responsibility applies to the personal contacts between health
service users and providers, the planning and provision of
services to populations, and the accountability of health workers
to those whose wealth they spend and whose lives they influence.

Professional-Patient Relationships

How can individuals share more responsibility for their use of
the health service with those who provide the care? How can we
develop the 'autonomy' advocated by the *Black Report*? At this
personal level our ideas of 'participation' and 'democracy' are
inadequate, for illness by its nature promotes dependence, and
dependence itself is a recurrent feature of social relationships.
No formula, concept or new practice can suddenly transform
habits and personality structures welded into the social
structure. When we think of professional relationships based on
mutual responsibility, we are thinking of changes occurring over
generations, and proceeding at different rates amongst different
groups of people. Children from poor, single-parent families in
sub-standard housing may carry their sense of hopelessness and
worthlessness long after their material and social circumstances
have improved, influencing their lives, health and use of health
services for decades. On the other hand, the workforce offered
regular personal health screening, or regular reviews of their
working environment, might change attitudes and practices
within a few years.

Changes will occur over long periods, will be bilateral, and
complex. For example, today a man wanting a medical
certificate to legitimise his prolonged absence from work
because of some minor complaint may meet a variety of
responses. A certificate and legitimacy, may be given to him. It
may be refused, forcing him into conflict with his employer if he
not able or willing to return to work. Or he may be asked if there
are other problems prompting his absence from work – illness in
the family, heavy drinking, depression, or another more ominous
symptom that he fears and hides. The way in which he and his
doctor respond will depend on their relationship, and the degree
to which they have developed a mutual understanding and

mutual criticism.

To give the certificate without enquiring about other problems may be sympathetic, but unhelpful. To refuse the certificate may be mistaken, and force an ill person to work prematurely, but it also reflects the professional's indifference to the patient's circumstances. To search for other, hidden problems may express an understanding that allows help to be given, or could appear as an unwarranted intrusion on privacy and self-respect. All of these options occur everyday, and are created by the varying relationships between people and health professionals. How can these options change? Sympathy is eesential in health care, but it can also be used instead of time and understanding, as a way of avoiding action. Indifference expresses the hostility the affluent and powerful so often feels towards supposed inferiors, but it may sometimes provoke reaction and stimulate change. Pursuit of hidden problems can create opportunities for better communication, but it can also be an expression of one person's control over another, a measure of dominance rather than equality. When relationships between professionals and the public are so complex, how can we promote shared responsibility for health care?

If there is an answer, it is through the clarification of roles. Is it a health worker's job to police sickness-absence from work, or should the NHS concentrate on that much greater problem of ill people continuing to work? If the 'patient' is given the responsibility for accounting for absence through illness, what rights should s/he have in return? 'Rights' are rarely discussed in the NHS, for they challenge the idea of professional control. A pregnant woman has a right to a midwife's help, and her new-born child will have the right to attention from midwives and health visitors for a short time. After that rights give way to resources.

Should that be changed, so that we all, as 'patients', have rights to screening for preventable or treatable illnesses, to fertility control (including easy, accessible abortion services) or to specialist help, in our own homes, when we are dying? 'Patients' Rights' might sound unexciting, but they would shift obligations onto health workers and responsibilities onto service users, in a way that market-based concepts of professional relationships cannot do. Deciding which services should be available as of right, and which according to resource-availability, makes priorities into a social and political issue, not a personal one. Debating priorities demands that information is available and understood, including personal information about health and illness. Knowing that more money is being spent on terminal care than on cardiac surgery in one Health District may be important politically, but its significance will increase if each individual knows his or her likely and imminent need for either service.

Why should we not have an assessment of our personal health, offered to us as part of an NHS service? Why should we not have responsibility for the main record of our health and illness, even if NHS staff retain their records too? Such changes would take resources, and time, and would be labour-intensive rather than capital-intensive. They would also test the resilience of professionalism, for how equal can doctor and patient be, when the former earns two, three or four times more than the latter, has a priviledged education, and probably comes from an affluent background?

Changing Methods of Work

On its own, however, increasing the availability and accessibility of professional advice could do more to satisfy wants than needs. The role of the health service is to direct professionals towards those needs, so that they introduce the health service's objectives to the population through the daily contacts between service users and service providers. The objective will need to be worked out, explained and pursued. Without public involvement none of this can occur. Enthusiastic professionals may urge that cervical cancer screening should be offered to women working at a particular enterprise, or living on a particular housing estate, and a responsive health service may set up a clinic. No-one will understand why women do not use the service, for no-one started out by asking the women whether they had had screening tests done elsewhere, or whether they wanted them, or how they thought they ought to be done. Rejected by those they aimed to help, the professionals may be tempted into cynical criticism of others' ignorance, or become responsive to lobbying from more articulate people with fewer needs but greater expectations. 'Need' had been seen as an academic issue, arising from local death rates from cervical cancer, the relative ease of detecting early malignant change, and the effectiveness of treatment.

This formula for meeting needs misses out the impact on the women's lives of ideas and expectations about illness and health, fears about medical intervention as well as about cancer, and the overlap between different parts of the NHS. The process of screening should begin with the first explanations of the reasoning behind it, and not with the first clinic appointments and the poster on the health centre notice-board. The public meetings, the questionnaires collected door-to-door, or the market-place canvass may give the most important information of all: that cervical cancer screenings have already been done, at work or in the antenatal and family-planning clinics; that the women want female not male staff; that few believe the problem is worth the effort.

When professionals are required to report on what they have done, to compare their work with their plans, and to alter activity according to changes in people's needs, they will alter the character of relationships between themselves and those they serve. Making sure that small children are developing normally, and are free from physical and mental impediments, takes time and good relations between health worker, parents and child. Most children develop normally, and the yield from all this effort is fairly small. To justify the sacrifice of time, the parents need to understand the rationale behind this surveillance; and the number of handicapped children, their degree of handicap, and their age when the handicap was recognised, need to be measured. Without explanation, the service is not utilised, and without measurement it cannot be improved accurately, nor can longer-term support be planned.

Convincing an individual with severe high blood pressure to accept long-term treatment for a symptomless condition requires the health worker to convey complex ideas about risks to a person more familiar with ideas of disease. It also demands proof that treatment is worthwhile and effective, and that requires the measurement of outcomes for whole populations over long periods of time. No-one can pretend that infrequent, brief, and perhaps impersonal contacts between health professionals and their patients can achieve these educative and evaluative tasks, yet the NHS as presently organised provides no more than that. Every person at risk from high blood pressure can be found, if we choose to do so, and advised. The outcome, in terms of rates of death or disability from strokes, heart attacks and kidney failure can be measured, to see how well or badly medical intervention works. All that activity requires understanding on the part of people using the service, and acceptance of obligations by professionals. Both understanding and obligations evolve, with minimal conflict, when both parties have responsibility for health care. Participatory democracy is not an option for management of health services, but a necessity when commercial pressures and consumer interests are excluded.

Controlling Mechanisms

The concept of participatory democracy should not be confused with ideas of 'patient power', or any further extension of pressure-group politics into health service administration. It is the antidote to consumerism in health care, for its presupposes the exclusion of the commercial interests that distort the provision of services, whilst emphasising the obligations of health workers and the responsibilities of the public. It depends on the evolution of an agreed order of priorities for development, worked out at national level by a Department of Health that works in public, not in secret. It requires local Health Authorities to match the national programme of priorities with their own order, to report on progress to their constituents and to explain results in public.

Unlike the command structure evolved in sixties and seventies, it is biased against professional and private interests, and in favour of popular representation. It represents an obligatory democracy, in which those running and providing the services are compelled to measure and react to public needs, whilst the public has some responsibility for the running of the service. The representation for people's different needs, and the introduction of representative democracy to NHS management will create new administrative structures as well as modify existing ones. What those structures will be, and how they will work, we cannot predict, but we can begin to develop their prototypes. Trade union collaboration inside the NHS, local government involvement in health Authorities and health care planning, extended CHC powers, and novel forms of management of local services all offer opportunities for change, and for the development of a new kind of health care.

Our experience of participatory democracy is limited. The labour movement has had a hand in fostering the cult of expertise, and in creating centralised administrative structures designed to control health care spending. 'Municipal socialism' survives as an undercurrent within Labour but retains old solutions, like local government control of health services, which provide only partial answers to current problems. Community Health Councils can involve people in healthy policy-making in the positive way, despite their lack of powers. The Thatcher administration came to dislike the CHCs partly because their participatory functions could encourage habits hostile to the market, and blur political differences. Conservatives on CHCs have been known to defend local health services against cuts, effectively in defiance of their own government, precisely because familiarity with real problems undermines partisan judgements. Labour responses have been cool, too, with CHCs reporting difficulty in recruiting trade union representation. Voluntary organisations, like Age Concern, MIND or the British Diabetic Association, act as vehicles for participatory democracy, yet remain outside the scope of labour movement's political concern. Patients' committees in general practice can be mechanisms for people to influence the character and range of health care, at local level, but have no priority in reformers' thinking and remain the products of exceptional professional initiative. Only the women's movement has been able to prompt a labour movement response, and then only around a single aspect of the issue of fertility control, the defence of the 1967 Abortion Act.

This is the weakest element in the left's approach to health politics. The right has the market relationship as its basic form of social organisation. So far Labour has concentrated on a different relationship, between state and citizen, that was designed to modify the market relationship. In the future it may not be able to gain much advantage from this approach, and will have to think again about social organisation and the role of the state. The development of participatory democracy now, in experimental ways, could inspire that new thinking, and shift the initiative in health politics further to the left than it has ever been before.

Bibliography

These are some of the books and pamphlets that I have found most useful as sources of ideas and information.

Aaronovitch, S., *The Road from Thatcherism*, Lawrence & Wishart, 1981.

Abel-Smith, B., *Value for Money in Health Services*, Heinemann, 1976.

Barnard, K. and Lee, K. (eds), *Conflicts in the National Health Service*, Croom Helm, 1977.

Brown, R.G.S., *The Changing National Health Service*, RKP, 1973.

Cartwright, F., *A Social History of Medicine*, Longman, 1977.

Cartwright, A., and Anderson, R., *General Practice Revisited*, Tavistock, 1981.

Greenwood, V. and Young, J., *Abortion On Demand*, Pluto Press, 1976.

Ham, C., *Health Policy in Britain*, Macmillan, 1982

Haywood, S. and Alaszewski, A., *Crisis in the Health Service*, Croom Helm, 1980.

Honigsbaum, F., *The division in British Medicine*, Kogan Page, 1979.

Hutt, A., *British Trade Unionism*, Lawrence & Wishart, 1975.

Kitzinger, S. and Davis, J. (eds), *The Place of Birth*, Oxford, 1978.

McKeown, T., *The Role of Medicine*, Blackwell, 1979.

Merrison, Sir Alec (chairman), *Report of the Royal Commission on the National Health Service*, HMSO, 1979.

Navarro, V., *Class Struggle, the State and Medicine*, Martin Robertson, 1978.

Navarro, V., *Medicine under Capitalism*, Croom Helm, 1976.

Politics of Health Group, *Going Private*, 1981.

Robson, J., *Quality, Inequality and Health Care*, Medicine in

Society (special edition), 1977.

Sethi, A. and Dimmock, S. (eds), *Industrial Relations and Health Services*, Croom Helm, 1982.

Sjostrom, H. and Nilsson, R., 'Thalidomide and the Power of the Drug Companies', Penguin, 1972.

Stacey, M. and Reid, M., *Health and the Division of Labour*, Croom Helm, 1977.

Stark Murray, D., *Blueprint for Health*, George, Allen & Unwin, 1973.

Stark Murray, D., *Why a National Health Service?*, Pemberton, 1971.

Townsend, P. and Davidson, N., *Inequalities in Health*, Penguin 1982

Tudor Hart, J., *The NHS in England and Wales*, Communist Party, 1974.

Watkin, B., *Documents on Health and Social Services*, Methuen, 1975

Glossary

AHA	Area Health Authority
ALRA	Abortion Law Reform Association
ASW	Association of Scientific Workers
ASTMS	Association of Scientific, Technical & Managerial Staffs
BMA	British Medical Association
BUPA	British United Provident Association
CHC	Community Health Council
CT	Computerised Tomography
COHSE	Confederation of Health Service Employees
DHA	District Health Authority
DHSS	Department of Health & Social Security
FPC	Family Practitioner Committee
GP	General Practitioner
GNCTU	General National Consolidated Trades Union
HSS	Hospital Scientific Service
IDT	Industrial Disputes Tribunal
JHDA	Junior Hospital Doctors Association
MPU	Medical Practitioners Union
MHIWU	Mental Hospital & Institutional Workers Union
MRC	Medical Research Council
NBPI	National Board for Prices & Incomes
NHI	National Health Insurance
NUPE	National Union of Public Employees
NMR	Nuclear Magnetic Resonance
NPHT	Nuffield Provincial Hospital Trust
PPP	Private Patients Plan
RAWP	Resource Allocation Working Party
RCGP	Royal College of General Practitioners
RCM	Royal College of Midwives
RCN	Royal College of Nursing
RHA	Regional Health Authority
SDP	Social Democratic Party
SEN	State Enrolled Nurse
SHA	Socialist Health Association (formerly SMA)

SMA	Socialist Medical Association
SMSA	State Medical Services Association
SRN	State Registered Nurse
TUC	Trades Union Congress
WPA	Western Provident Association

Index